WAVE HANDS LIKE CLOUDS

D1611334

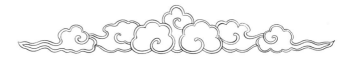

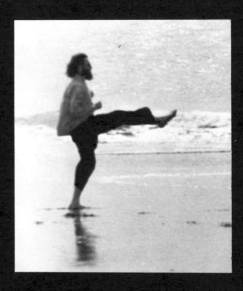

The clouds pass and the rain does its work, and all individuals flow into their forms.

I Ching: Hexagram I. The Creative

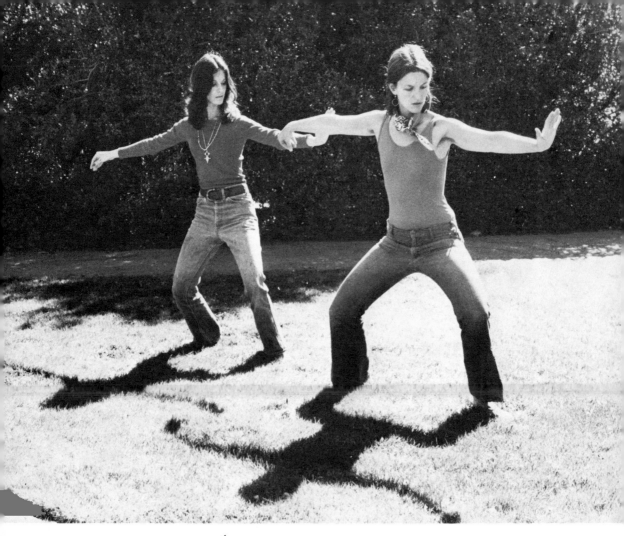

A Chinese Yoga of Meditation in Motion

KUNG FU   INNER TRUTH

KUANG PING TAI CHI

WAVE HANDS LIKE CLOUDS

BY LI PO & ANANDA

Credits and Acknowledgments

*Grateful acknowledgment is made for permission to reprint the poem
"Empty Infinity" on p. 41 from* The Secret of the Golden Flower, A
Chinese Book of Life, *translated into German and explained by Richard
Wilhelm; English translation by Cary F. Baynes. Reprinted by permission
of Harcourt Brace Jovanovich, Inc.*

Lines from the I Ching: Or Book of Changes, *translated by Richard
Wilhelm, rendered into English by Cary F. Baynes, Bollingen Series XIX
(copyright © 1950, 1967 by the Bollingen Foundation), reprinted by permission of Princeton University Press.*

Photography and design: Ananda
Special pictures: Sanje
Copy editors: Beverly Terwoman, Denny Wiseman, Margaret Cheney
*Other Contributors: The authors are grateful to many people who helped
along the way.*

Library of Congress Cataloging in Publication Data
Ananda.
    Wave hands like clouds.
    Bibliography: p.
    1. T'ai chi ch'uan. I. Po, Li, joint author.
II. Title.
GV481.P58 1975   796.8'159   75–9351
ISBN 0–06–121650–X pbk.

10 9 8 7 6 5 4 3

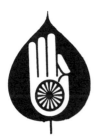

BAMBOO PUBLISHING
P. O. Box 1037
Ft. Bragg, CA. 95437

We dedicate this work to Kuanyin,

Merciful, Compassionate Bodhisattva,

She Who Listens to the Cries of the World!

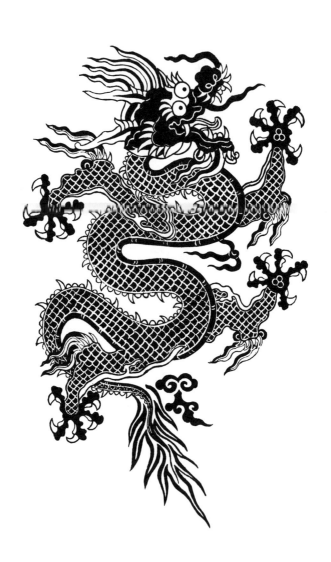

CONTENTS

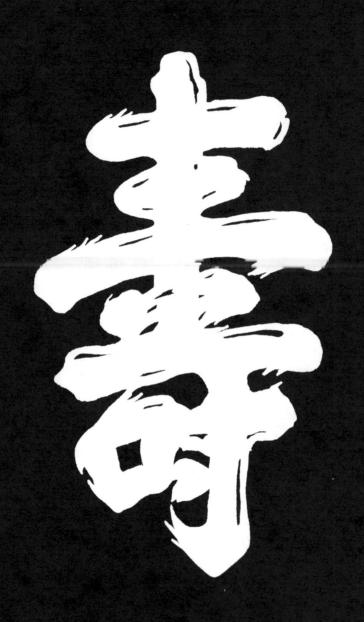

FOREWORD

This book is the outgrowth of our students' requests for a training manual. It is a "how to do it" book of Tai Chi. There is basic information of general interest about Tai Chi—what it is, its history explained, and how to perform it, in detail. Contained here is a complete manual of the Kuang Ping Tai Chi form—with pictures, clearly self-instructional in nature. They were posed by the authors and their friends.

Included also is a complete perpetuating system for body health and continuous psycho-physical development. Kuang Ping Tai Chi is unusual. It has been introduced to the United States quite recently, while the other systems of Yang style Tai Chi have been taught here since 1937. Kuang Ping instruction began in San Francisco in 1964. It originated in the region of Honan Province in North China. The body positions encourage development of supple, flexible physique with deep, open leg positions and full extensions of arms and legs. Kuang Ping Tai Chi is performed with broad steps and well-bent knees. It is a difficult Tai Chi to perform effortlessly, until the legs and lower back become strong and developed. However, when performed gracefully, it is extraordinarily beautiful.

Interest in Kuang Ping Tai Chi is growing, and we hope this book will help people to learn it with joyfulness.

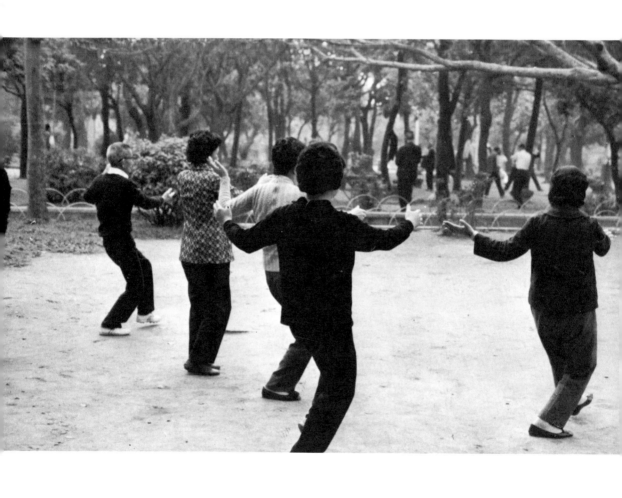

WHAT IS TAI CHI

Tai Chi is a system of physical exercise and a way of moving meditation which has been part of daily life in China for centuries. The Chinese characters for Tai Chi mean Supreme Ultimate. The Tai Chi movement patterns were derived from forms for self-defense.

As a system of physical exercise the benefits Tai Chi offers are similar to those from hatha yoga. Performance imparts a sense of well-being and physical stimulation. It improves health.

As moving meditation, it helps the individual to progress along the path of self-knowledge. From Tai Chi, health and energy are acquired for sustained concentration. Meditation helps to develop inner strength, confidence, and personal efficiency. We grow and change, remaining open.

Tai Chi is also an art form, an alchemical practice, and a ritual dance. It becomes personal art when the pattern is thoroughly mastered and remembered. When thoughts are not directed to anticipating what comes next, there is absorption in the quiet beauty of Tai Chi and the shapes the performer makes in space.

Tai Chi is alchemical because we utilize the elements in

the atmosphere to transform ourselves. When we perform Tai Chi, we absorb oxygen, heat, and light and convert them to fire and water. It is ritual dance, practiced daily. It makes us become radiant!

When practiced as self-defense, it is called Tai Chi Chuan. Chuan is Chinese for fist. Tai Chi teaches us to be yielding, nonresistant, and nonviolent. We learn not to meet force with force, but to interpret energy by the practice of Tui Sho, pushing hands.

Tui Sho is used as a training method for two people who learn to work together in a supportive way, learning and applying Tai Chi defense movements. There is no value in disciplining the mind and the body for physical violence of any kind. At the same time, there are some basic elementary principles of self-defense that are useful in evading or nullifying an attack, should it be necessary. Perhaps once in your life someone might try to commit an aggression against you. At that time you must be able to stop it. Tai Chi is helpful in learning how to get out of the way, quickly.

Techniques of self-defense need to be practiced thoroughly to be directly useful. Physical demonstrations and training with a teacher are best for learning practical applications. Since actual conditions of real attacks cannot be anticipated, it is futile to program ourselves heavily with theoretical defenses. Therefore, the best application of Tai Chi is as a physical meditation program. The Pushing Hands formulas were developed to teach sensitivity to an opponent's force, rather than as direct applications of a technique. Although some schools have developed sets for two people incorporating uses, such theoretical programming does not lead to personal liberation.

*Tai Chi is also called **Kung Fu**. Lately these words have become popularized. People believe that **Kung Fu** means fast fighting movements originated by the Chinese. The character for study or work is **Kung**; **Fu** means person. **Kung Fu** is any task which requires time, patience, and study. Tai Chi in that sense is **Kung Fu**.*

Literature Study

*The **I** Ching and the **Tao Teh Ching** are the ancient philosophical works that are studied with Tai Chi. These books contain the roots of the three major ideologies of China—Confucianism, Taoism, and Buddhism. Within the **I** Ching, the sixty-first hexagram is entitled "Chung Fu." This hexagram is called "Inner Truth." It is also called the **Kung Fu** hexagram.*

> *Inner Truth indicates a heart free of prejudices and therefore open to the truth.**

It is with this idea that practice and study of Tai Chi should be undertaken.

* *I Ching,* trans. Richard Wilhelm, p. 235.

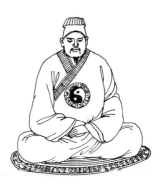

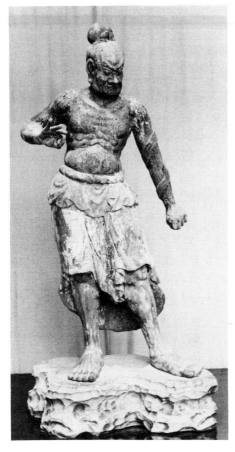

A BRIEF History

In ancient times, Tai Chi was named "Chang Chuan," long boxing, "San Shih Chi," and the thirteen forms. The roots of Chinese physical culture systems are buried in a period known as "wild" or unverifiable history, so that an accurate chronology is at best only probable. Early documents refer to a surgeon named Hua-t'o (born A.D. 190), who taught a series of exercises based on the movements of animals. But even before this, in the time of Confucius, slow, graceful exercises based on animal movements were performed.

Since its origin, Tai Chi has passed through many changes and variations. If ever there was a time when the forms were standardized, it certainly is not today. Tai Chi systems have many styles, as they must always have had, even when practiced within the monasteries by monks.

The Famous Legend of Chang San Fung

Tai Chi was created in the fourteenth century by a Taoist monk, Chang San Fung. Master Chang witnessed a fight between a bird and a snake in which the bird kept trying to spear the snake with its beak. The snake, through flexible circular movements, *was able to evade every thrust. The fight lasted several days and each combatant continued through flexible maneuvering and soft evasive countering. Eventually the snake caught the bird by ensnaring it in its coils. This showed Chang that a hard, strong opponent could be subdued by a less physically forceful, but more clever, strategy.*

Contemporary Tai Chi is the method of body training passed on to us from the Chen family of Honan, who are said to have learned Master Chang San Fung's forms. Chen Wang Ting and Chiang Fa helped the Chen family improve their hard style of Kung Fu and taught by using soft, gentle training methods. Since then, each generation of Chen masters has been improving, changing, and developing forms and training practices. The later Yang and Wu schools of Tai Chi are also variants of Chen training.

In China today there are many methods of physical culture based on the original, old practices of Taoist-Buddhist monastic centers. The Indian monk Damo brought yoga from India to China in the fifth century. His I Chin Ching (Muscle Change Classic) exercises were taught to monks to enable them to undergo a long day of prayer, fasting, and meditation.

Although some Taoist adepts and Buddhist monks were trained in martial arts, boxing and weapon forms were undertaken mainly by military and ruling classes, quite apart from the teachings of religion. Some warriors, repelled by the application of their deadly arts, would often retreat from the world to stay in monasteries, after they had seen the futility of battle.

The training method of Tai Chi in this book is from Yang

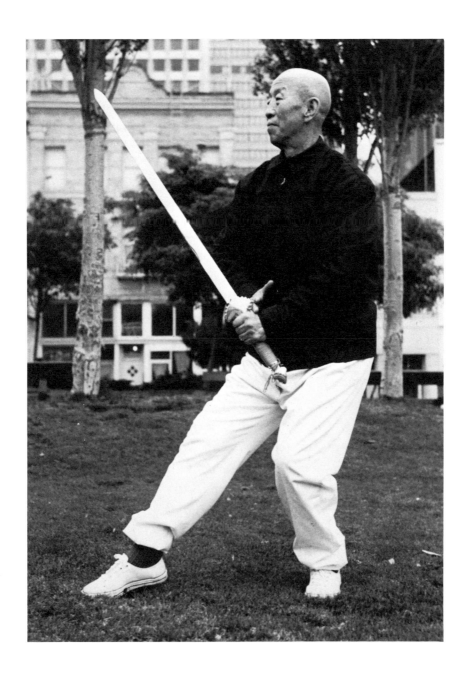

Pan Hou, first son of Yang Lu Chan. It was Yang Lu Chan who first learned from the Chen family. Long ago, Tai Chi was practiced secretly and not taught freely. Yang sought employment in the Chen household as a servant in order to spy on the family Tai Chi practice. His talent in learning through watching became known to the family later on and they agreed to teach him.

One day an unknown boxer came to Honan to challenge the leading Chen masters, who were away. The unknown challenger nevertheless fought and defeated those of the family who were able to compete with him. At last he agreed to try out Yang, who was only a servant and not really eligible to compete. But the family had already lost face, so there was no further harm in one more loss. Yang surprised everyone by winning the match and redeeming the family honor. Because of this victory, Yang was formally accepted as a Chen trainee.

Yang Pan Hou, first son of Yang Lu Chan, taught his servant, Wong, who later retired to a monastery outside Peking. It was there that our teacher, Kuo Lien Ying, then a young man, went to challenge the ex-servant. Wong, at 112 years of age, was able to stop all Kuo's attempts to defeat him. Following this incident, Kuo studied with Master Wong for many years. Wong lived to the age of 123.

发展体育运动

增强人民体质

毛泽东

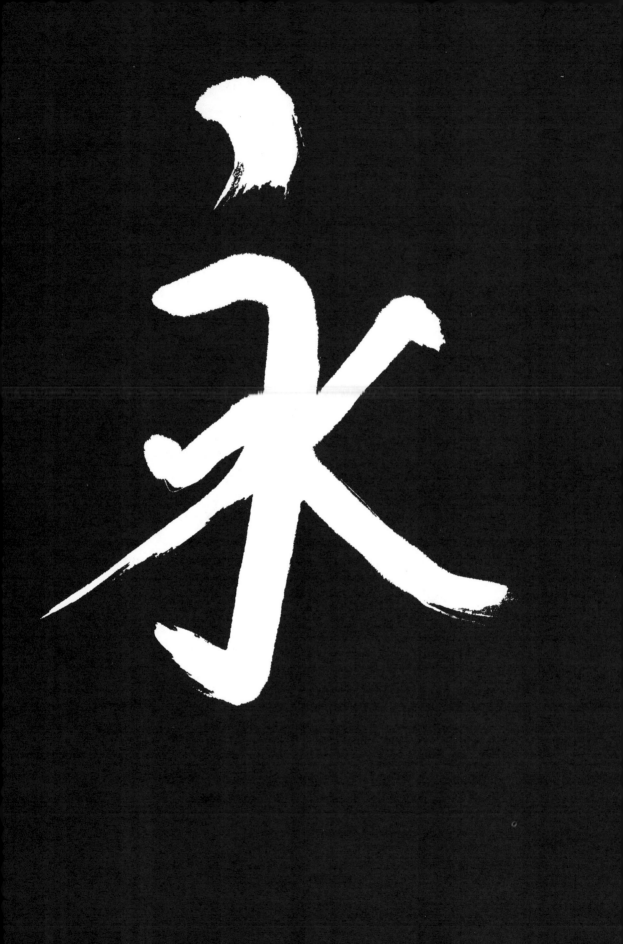

WARMUP
EXERCISES

How to Begin

The warmup exercises which follow have been in use in China for centuries and form a system for self-directed study. They are totally noncompetitive. Still performed today in China and Taiwan, they are classified as Internal System *exercises. They are practiced slowly and consciously, with particular attention to the incoming and outgoing breaths. They provide gentle stimulation and massage to the internal organs, as well as the joints, ligaments and nerves. There is no emphasis on muscular development or exertion of physical strength.*

Traditionally, the exercises have been used to prevent and cure arthritic conditions by dissolving impurities that have been deposited at the joints. Internal System *exercises help develop strong nerves and produce mental energy.*

External Systems are exercise systems using muscular force. That includes many modern sports and activities. The Internal System is meditation training. With slow, natural breathing the mind focuses on the body's movement. When your hand goes out, you observe it attentively. Your training stills the mind and keeps it from wandering, during practice and afterward.

Practice Tai Chi preliminary warmups before you perform the Tai Chi form. They loosen the body and help you maintain steadiness. If there is pain when performing these, stop the exercise and try it again some other time.

The Movement of Force

Although no moving steps are taken during the rotating exercises which follow, there is body movement. It is helpful to visualize the path of the movement as a spiraling action. The spiral motion winds and recurs starting at the toes and flowing through the spine, moving all the joints.

Waist Rotations

Stand erect with both feet close together. Place the palms on your back next to each other. Point the fingers downward, hands touching and positioned at the back of the waist (lumbar vertebrae). Without moving your head, push the torso forward and move it all the way to the right and spiral around and around, clockwise. Repeat the rotations about 32 times and change the direction of the rotations to counter-clockwise. In the process of performing this exercise, don't lock your knees at the joints; keep them loose so they can spiral. These rotations exercise the joints, while providing massage to the internal organs. If you exert gentle pressure with your hands on your back, you will be massaging the spinal nerves and kidneys.

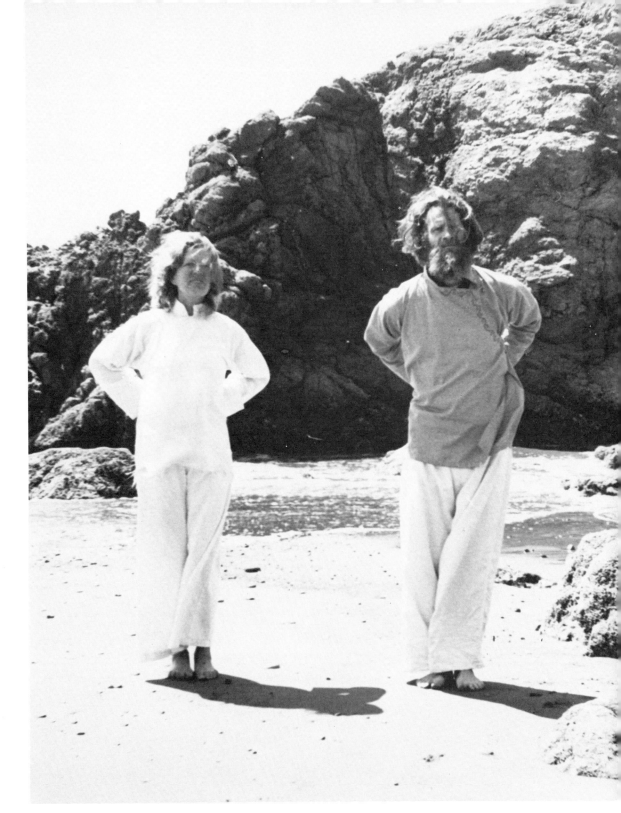

Hip Rotations

Stand erect and place both feet apart with the distance of one footprint between them. Keep your feet parallel and facing front. Keep your toes front. Place your hands on your hip bones. Perform spiral rotations with your hips as follows: Swing the hips straight across to the right as far as they will go and then shift the hips to the rear. Then push the hips forward. Continue swinging the hips to the right and to the rear in clockwise rotations. After 32 repetitions change the swing of the hips to the left, then the rear, making counter-clockwise rotations. There are two aims to this exercise—first to loosen the hip joints, and second to stimulate the internal organs.

Knee Circling

Place both feet together and bend your knees. Place the palms on your knee caps. Make circles with your knees. Perform this circling 8 times clockwise and 8 times counter-clockwise. The number of repetitions is optional and can be increased if desired. Knee circling is helpful in strengthening knees and ankles.

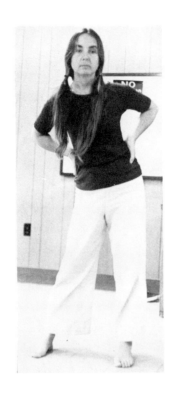

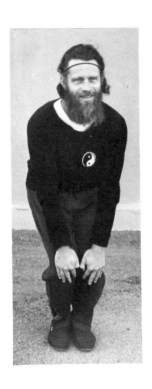

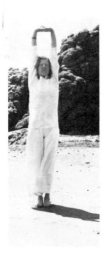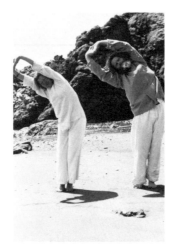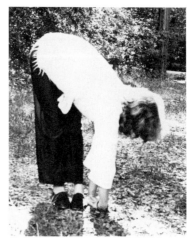

Monkey Stretches Upward and Downward

Stand erect with feet together. Interlace your fingers and keep them interlaced for the entire exercise. Stretch both arms straight overhead, keeping the elbows close to your ears and pushing upward toward the sky. Then slowly sway from side to side, bending at the waist. Repeat these side bends several times. Then extend your arms straight forward, bending at the waist and bringing the palms down (fingers still interlaced) to touch the ground. Don't bend your knees, and try to gaze upward so you get a good stretch in back of your neck and under your chin. Remain in this position without movement for a few moments, until the breath flows naturally.

When there is no difficulty in touching the ground (don't force it; it will happen if you persevere), proceed a bit further and twist the waist all the way to the left, moving your palms left, on the ground. Next, turn to the right, touching the ground with palms on the right. These movements stretch and twist your spine.

If you had trouble touching the ground, try bending forward without moving up and down, merely remaining with bent waist for a few moments. Then swing your arms to and fro for a few moments.

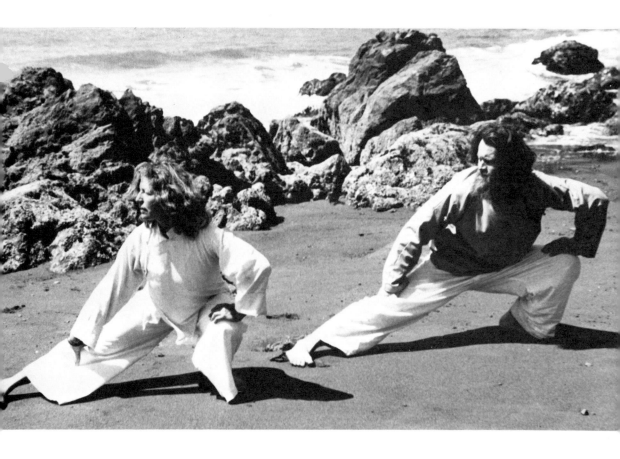

Tiger Crouches Downward

Stand erect and separate your feet to a distance slightly wider than your shoulders. Bend your knees, keeping feet parallel, actually toeing in slightly. Place your palms on your kneecaps, right hand on right knee and left hand on left knee. Bend the right knee deeply, squatting down and bringing all your body weight to the right side. Try to keep your spine erect. Don't bend forward to compensate for bending downward. Keep the heels firmly rooted to the ground. Now shift all the weight to the left side and bend your left knee, straightening the right knee and squatting to the left. This exercise strengthens the legs, while stretching the lower back and the insides of the thighs.

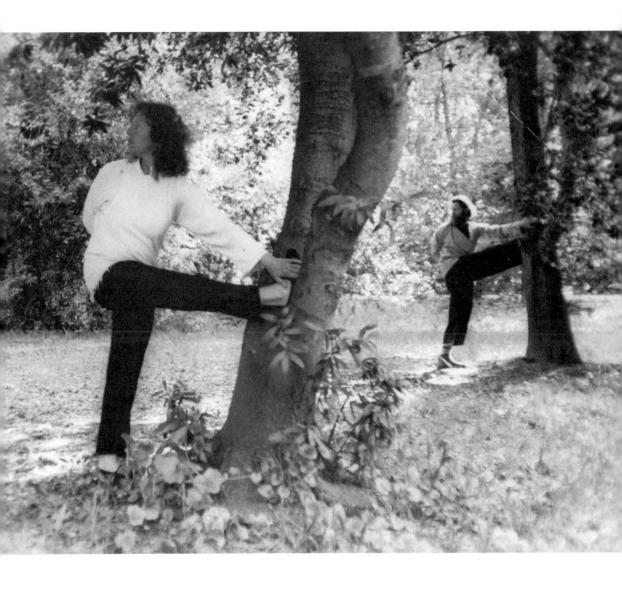

Leg Stretches

Raise either leg as shown and rest it on the edge of a table or window ledge. Point your toe toward your face so that the heel stretches. The supporting foot should face front and not turn

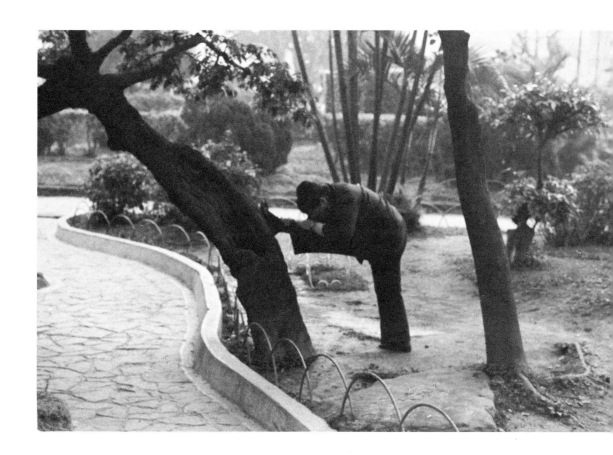

out. Bend forward, leading with your chin. See pictures for placement of hands. Turn your head around, trying to see directly behind. Perform this exercise on each leg. This type of stretching is designed to lengthen the hamstrings. Caution is essential. Should it hurt you, stop at once. This is a gradual exercise where a sign of pain means "stop."

After the above, bend at the waist and bring your face forward, trying to touch your chin to your toe. This exercise is preparation for the one which follows.

Phoenix Eating Its Ashes

Stand erect and step forward with either leg. Place the extended leg on its heel with the toe pointing up. Bend forward and down, stretching from the waist. Bend the back knee deeply and keep all weight on the back leg. Reach forward with both hands to grasp the outstretched foot. Try to bring the chin forward, attempting to touch your chin to the toes of your outstretched foot.

This is the most difficult of the exercises given so far. It is not impossible to achieve. The Chinese tell the story of the phoenix: it falls to its death into flames and rises up again, reborn. When you can touch your chin to your toes, you will feel reborn, like the phoenix.

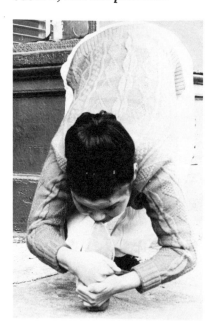

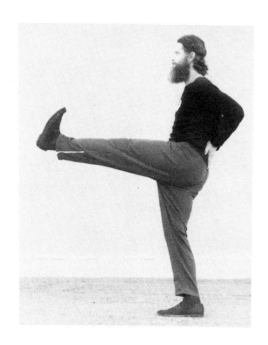

Diagonal Leg Raises

Place your hands on your lower back, at the lumbar vertebrae. Step left and forward (diagonally) with the left foot and raise the right foot up to the left, straightening it completely. Extend your heel and point the toes inward toward the body. Continuing, step forward and right with the right foot and raise up the left foot, thrusting it to the right. Extend the heel, while pointing the toes toward the body.

Perform these walking leg raises slowly and repeat, taking about 20 steps with each foot. Practice develops balance and coordination.

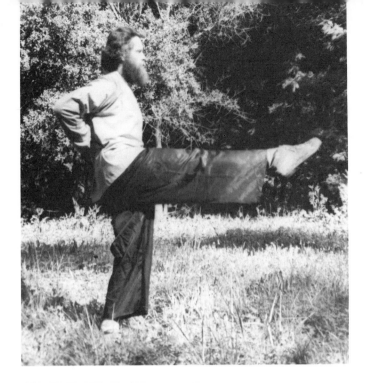

Straight Leg Raises

Stand erect and imagine that you are about to walk a tightrope. Place your hands on your lower back, as in the exercise above. Step straight forward with the right foot, raising the left foot up as high as possible and point the toe. Bring the leg slowly down and put it on the ground about a foot length in front of you on the imaginary tightrope. Transfer all weight onto it and raise the right leg, pointing it as before and stepping forward. Repeat about 20 steps for each foot.

Both the Diagonal Leg Raises and the Straight Leg Raises are training exercises for kicking, but they are performed as slow leg movements, rather than as fast kicks. Slow movements require more concentration than quick ones and the effects on the body are better. You develop conscious control. Fast body action often causes quick contraction, and muscular stiffness results. Injuries can occur when performing exercises without conscious attention.

In the Internal Systems *(Tai Chi, Shing Yee, Pa Kua) the emphasis is on slow performance and careful training to develop mind-body control.*

MORE Chinese Exercises

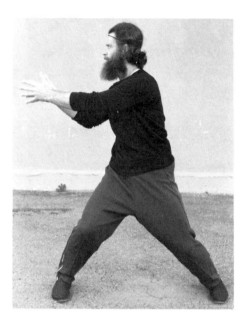 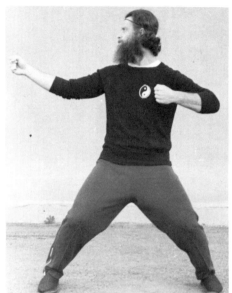

Draw the Bow

Assume the Horse posture, see page 35. Maintain bent knees for the entire exercise. Turn the waist to the left and extend both hands to the left, palms facing each other. Open and stretch your fingers as widely as possible. Now the hands become fists and "draw the bow" by bringing the right fist to the right, the left fist to the left, exerting a moment of tension at the end. Continuing, turn your body at the waist to the right and extend both arms to the right, and continue, as if drawing a giant bow. Repeat about 20 times.

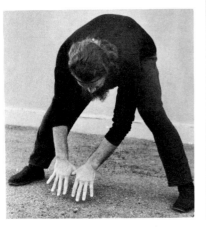 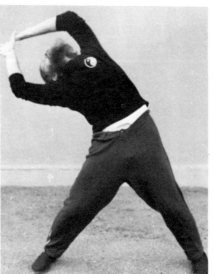 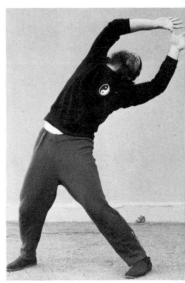

Sea Serpent Riding the Waves

Assume the Horse posture, page 35. The knees are bent during the entire maneuver. Raise the arms overhead and bend your waist forward, dropping your head and arms toward the left knee. Now swing the head and arms to the right and return to the Horse posture, raising and stretching the arms upward and backward. Shift your waist to the left and drop your head and arms again, beginning the circling as before. Thus far, counter-clockwise circling has been described. Repeat this circling 8 times and then stretch your arms upward and to the center to stabilize yourself and your breathing. Continue this exercise moving clockwise by dropping the head and arms to the right and begin clockwise circling for 8 repetitions. This will provide a good spinal stretch and help develop balance.

Backbends

In the Horse posture (page 35), place your hands, palms to-gether, on the lumbar vertebrae. Bend the knees deeply and push your hips forward. Continue bending backward, reaching upward with your arms, and move them back and down as far as you can. Repeat several times, approximately 8 or more.

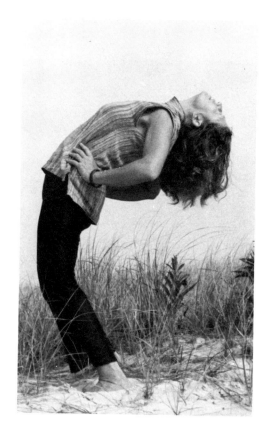

The Wheel

Begin in the Horse posture (page 35) again, and raise the arms overhead, reaching backward gradually and going lower and lower until reaching the ground with your palms. The advanced posture is practiced with your toes touching the ground and the shoulders above one finger of each hand.

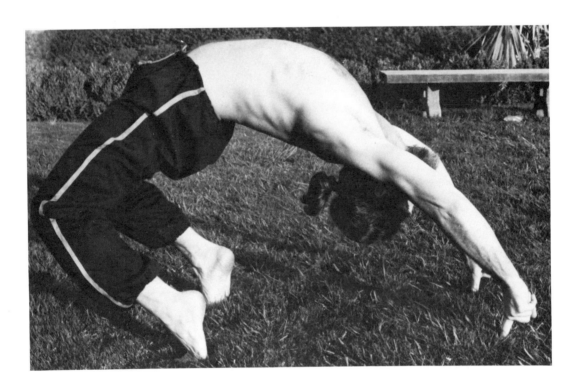

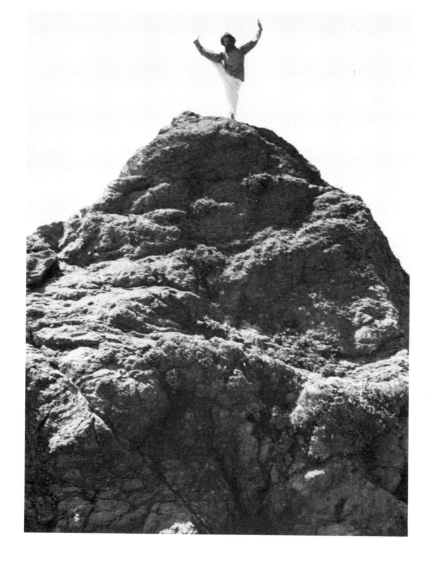

Full Scale

Starting with an erect body, raise the right leg with the right arm as high as it will go, remaining calmly balanced on the left foot. Perform this exercise with each leg.

Needle Scale

Lean forward and continue moving downward until the forehead touches the shin of the supporting leg. Extend the other leg fully overhead. Both hands grasp the ankle of the supporting leg. (Not illustrated.)

The Split

Kneel on one knee (back leg). Extend the front leg and stretch it out completely, bringing both the legs into complete contact with the ground. It's easier than you might think! Be careful when trying. If it hurts, stop immediately.

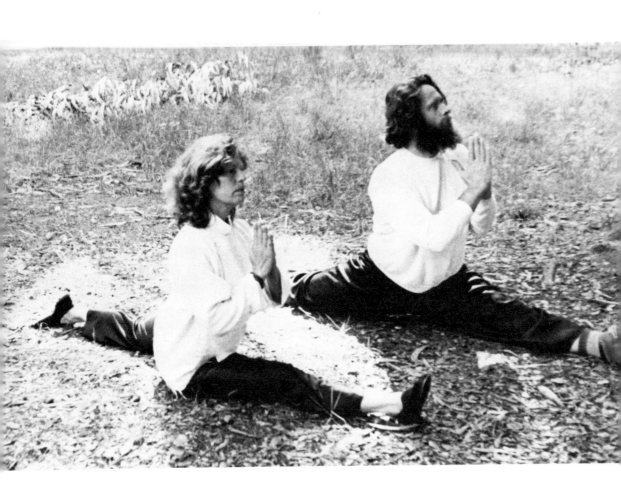

STANDING MEDITATION POSTURES

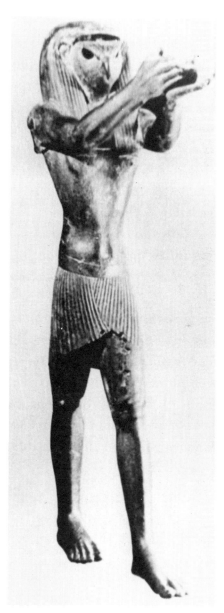

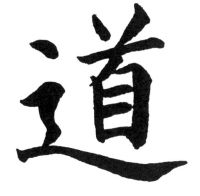

Universal Post

Relax and stand erect. Take a step forward with either foot. The size of the step is one footprint. Bend the forward leg at the knee and raise the heel off the ground one-quarter inch. Raise both arms to shoulder height and bend the elbows so that the arms are extended in a circle. Shift your body around, turning toward the forward leg so that the space between the hands falls directly over the extended leg. The fingers are open, curved and loose. All body weight is on the back leg. The front leg acts as a balancing point.

This is a healing posture which also develops strength and tranquility. Stand in a quiet place, preferably outdoors beside a tree. Let all thoughts go—allowing them to float away as if on a calm sea. Keep your eyes open, eyelids half closed, fixing the gaze on a distant place like the horizon or the endless sky. Watch your breathing by following the incoming breath and following the outgoing breath. Duration of practice should be 5 or 10 minutes for beginners. Gradually lengthen the time of practice to 15 minutes. Advanced students often stand in Universal Post 45 minutes to one hour each day. It's a good way to conclude morning practice.

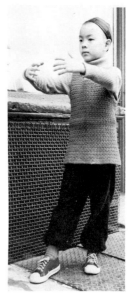

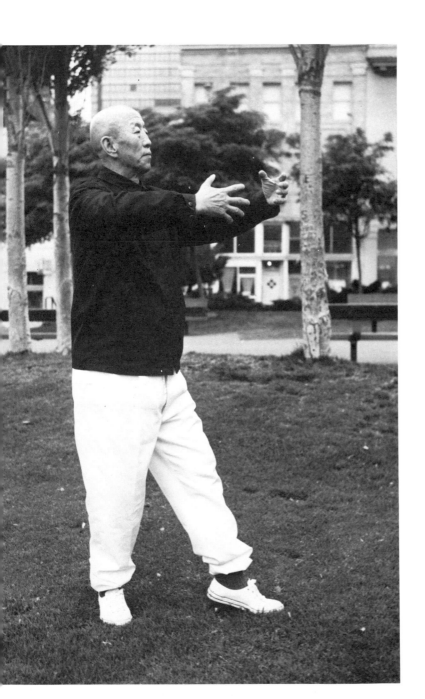

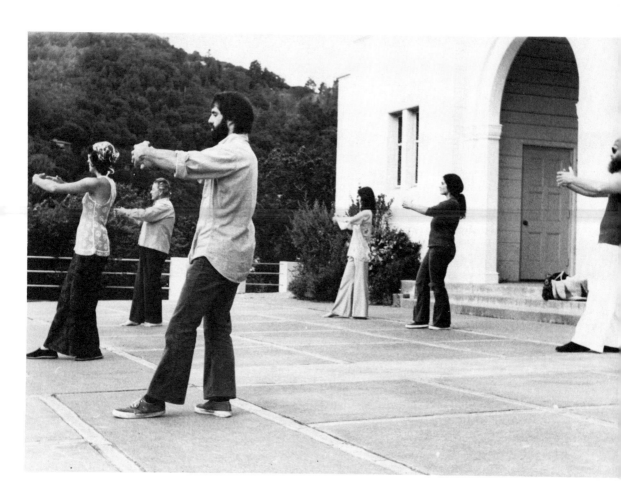

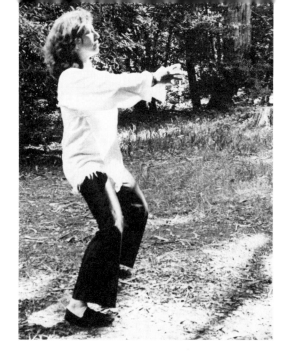

The Horse

Relax and stand erect. Spread your legs to a comfortable distance, slightly wider than the shoulders. Bend your knees and keep your feet turned to the front and well rooted to the ground. The spine is as erect as possible; the buttocks are pushed forward. The bent knees align over the toes. Raise your arms to chest height and let the fingers meet in the center, making a circle with your arms. Beginner's practice is 3 to 5 minutes, maintaining the Horse without external movement.

The Horse as a meditation posture is usually recommended by instructors for Shaolin, not for Tai Chi training. Instructors for Tai Chi claim that the Horse causes double-weightedness in the legs, which would be detrimental to a boxer. A Tai Chi boxer is trained to be stable with all or most weight on one leg at a time, rather than equally divided on two, for maximum agility and speed.

The Horse is an excellent healing posture. It induces relaxation, while developing stability and patience. The authors have seen a person with a stroke, and consequent paralysis of the right side, regain the use of his stricken limbs after patient, daily practice of standing in the Horse. He was practicing under the guidance of a well-known teacher.

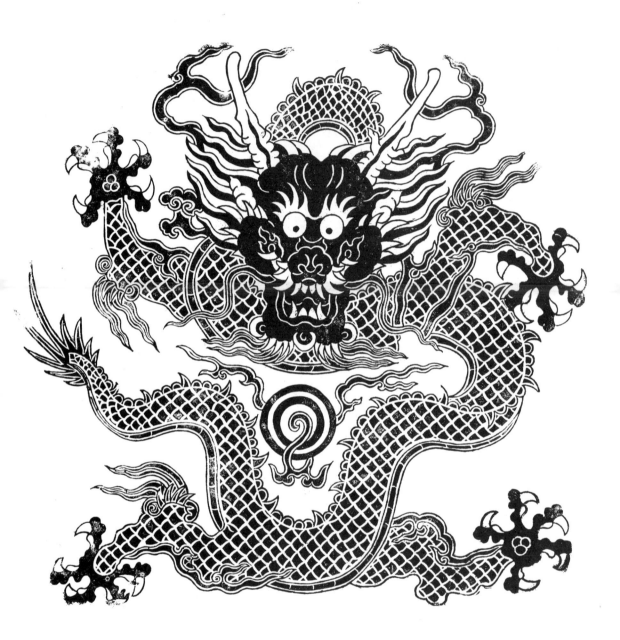

MEDITATION

Meditation is the direct experience of conscious awareness. It is knowledge of being at one with oneself, hence with the arrangement of nature. This kind of understanding bypasses thinking. It is intuitive knowledge acquired through practice and permeates the unconscious mind (beneath the threshold). It extends itself to the conscious mind by yielding a sense of well-being to the person who meditates. It is wisdom gained from integrating the different masks of personality—physical, emotional, intellectual, and spiritual.

Inner peace, relaxation, and joyfulness become known to the meditator and are the fruits of the labor. Meditation is work done joyfully. With Tai Chi meditation practice there is continuous development of awareness on many levels. It is waking up from lethargy to infinite energy.

Specifically for Tai Chi, there is one standing posture for meditation—it is Universal Post, described earlier. However, it does not matter what posture is used for meditation. Sitting comfortably in a chair, or cross-legged on a round cushion, or in Lotus Posture, or in Adept's Posture, are also used by many people. Whether sitting or standing, there must be

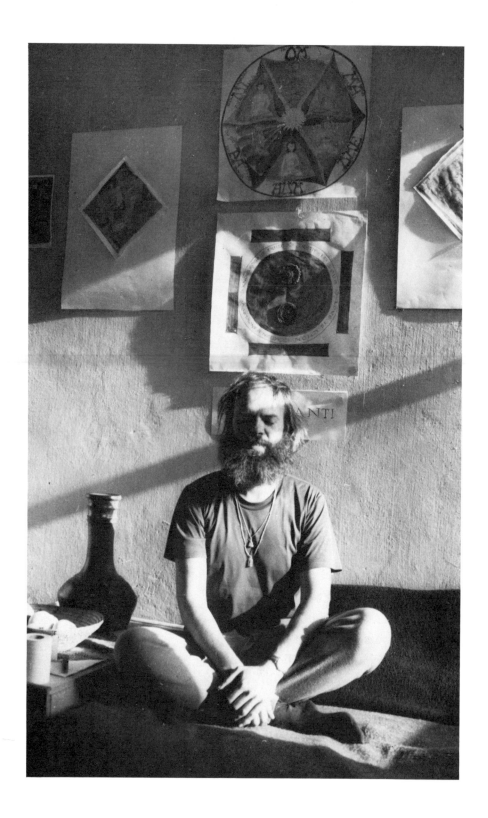

an erect spine and the wish to develop one-pointed concentration. While the mind is at rest the person meditating must not
be asleep or dozing.

So how do we actually meditate? What's going on inside our
heads and bodies, and what do we do about it?

To begin, we make a conscious effort to clear the mind of
all thoughts because they interfere with concentration. But
thoughts are persistent and we must deal with them. An effec-
tive way to handle thoughts is to let them pass through us, as
though they are moving clouds. We get a quick look at urgent
thoughts and can cope with them with increased vigor after
meditation. They will be taken care of. Just breathe. Follow
the incoming breath; follow the outgoing breath; full attention
on the incoming breath; full attention on the outgoing breath.
This is one-pointed concentration. It is also called fixation.
From this, meditation follows.

When the breath becomes stable, the meditator can engage in the practice of circulating the light within. This is
done by sending the attention to the top of the head, to the
crown, also called Sahasrara Chakra (by yogis), or thousand
petal lotus, and circulating light downward, permeating every
organ and every cell. Then return the light upward, to the
crown, and begin again. The duration of this procedure is
variable with each person. One pass can take a minute or five
minutes. As one circulates the light, one is engaged in healing
the body. All body processes function more slowly during meditation practice. Relaxation follows, as well as improved be-
havior. For a fuller discussion of the light within see The

Secrets of Chinese Meditation *by Lu K'uan Yu.*

There are, of course, myriad variations on the procedure given above, which happens to be Buddhist. It is often practiced with closed eyes, though Zen meditators keep eyes half shut (to let the light in), but focused about three feet ahead. Meditation is part of the daily ritual in Buddhist countries, as well as of yogis throughout the world. The Chinese Taoist method incorporates an additional concentration center—the Tan Tien. *The light is circulated from the crown and makes contact with the Tan Tien, also called the* cauldron *or* crucible. *The Tan Tien is located slightly below your navel. The yogis call this place the* Swadhisthana Chakra.

> *The circulation of light is a bathing or washing procedure—rising, inhaling and washing—contacting heaven (the crown) and descending, exhaling and bathing—contacting earth, continuing the circulation upward again.*

This is meditation practice for Tai Chi. It is also referred to as circulating the chi.

Empty Infinity

Without beginning, without end,
Without past, without future.
A halo of light surrounds the world of the law.
We forget one another, quiet and pure, altogether powerful and
      empty.
The emptiness is irradiated by the light of the heart and of heaven.
The water of the sea is smooth and mirrors the moon in its surface.
The clouds disappear in blue space; the mountains shine clear.
Consciousness reverts to contemplation; the moon disk rests alone.

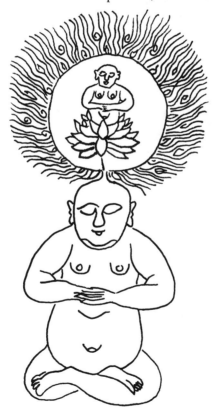

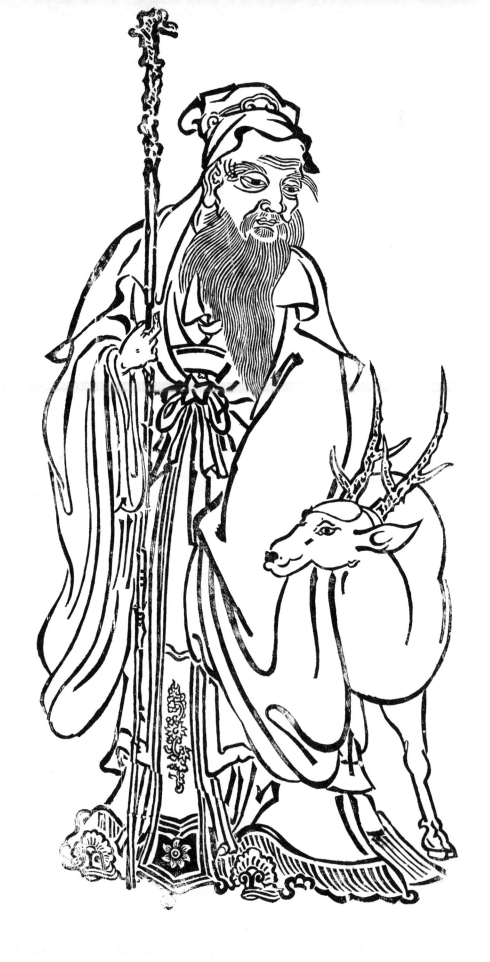

太極拳

TAI CHI CHUAN

TAI CHI:

A MANUAL OF FORM

How to Perform Tai Chi

Tai Chi movement is slow, continuous, and flowing, like performing ballet steps in water. Imagine that you're dancing in outer space, weightlessly. You are floating in air, with just the tiniest bit of air resistance against your body—like a leaf being carried by a gentle breeze.

Tai Chi is performed without exertion. The actions should be free of strain. Muscular exertion produces straining and inhibits the natural freedom of the body. Muscular exertion produces tension. We have been programmed since early childhood to "try hard." But trying hard makes us work against ourselves and inhibits our learning with ease. Tai Chi is moving meditation, to be practiced with both relaxation and concentration. Tai Chi begins as a structure but, when assimilated, it becomes a personal ritual.

Relaxed, natural movements come about when they are coordinated with the breath; when it stops and becomes irregular, you should become aware and allow it to flow smoothly. When the breath flows uninterruptedly, easy and effortless steps follow it.

Tai Chi breathing is low, with abdominal expansion, rather than high up in the chest and throat. The Tan Tien, the concentration point slightly below the navel, is the central focus for the breath. It is the chi storage point and the center of gravity. Imagine that the breath is a steady stream of light being inhaled at the Tan Tien and circulating throughout the entire body to the top of the head and back to the Tan Tien, extending to fingertips and toes. With patience and awareness your breath will circulate freely, without stoppages, and it will show in graceful, connected movements.

Before taking the first step in the Tai Chi set, take two full breaths in and out and again in and out—clearing your mind of all extraneous thoughts and your body of all obstacles. Focus full attention entirely upon yourself. Raise your tongue to the upper palate and keep it there during practice.

In Tai Chi, there are several recurring stances. Try to understand these postures and aim for ease in their fulfillment. Try also to practice the warmup exercises beforehand, as they are good preparation for steady breathing and concentration.

Posture

The spine is erect, the hips are forward, and the head is positioned as if suspended from above by a golden thread. The neck is straight; the chest natural, not expanded. All the joints are loose and moving freely. Special attention should be given to keeping the shoulders relaxed and the waist moving freely, without strain. The eyes follow the movement of the forward hand. When the gaze is coordinated with the hand movement, Tai Chi becomes expressive and graceful.

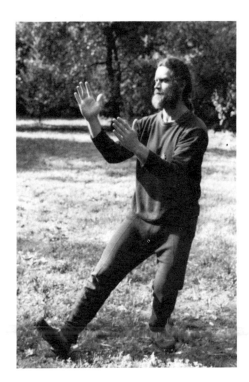
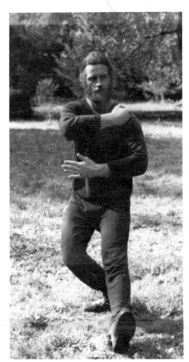

Basic Stances and Footwork

The feet move slowly and continuously, in an even, soft tempo. The center of gravity alternates from one foot to the other throughout the Tai Chi form. Remember that the knees are to be bent throughout. There are no straight-legged, erect postures.

T Steps

In a T step the feet are at a 90-degree angle to each other. The first time this occurs in the Tai Chi pattern is in Press Forward and Push, paragraph 3 of the Form (see page 51). The right foot takes a very wide and deep step to the right, placing the heel down first. T steps are performed with either foot stepping out, as described above and as in Single Whip, paragraph 5, the Form, page 52. Align your feet in a right angle; the heel of the stepping foot aligns with the instep of the stationary foot.

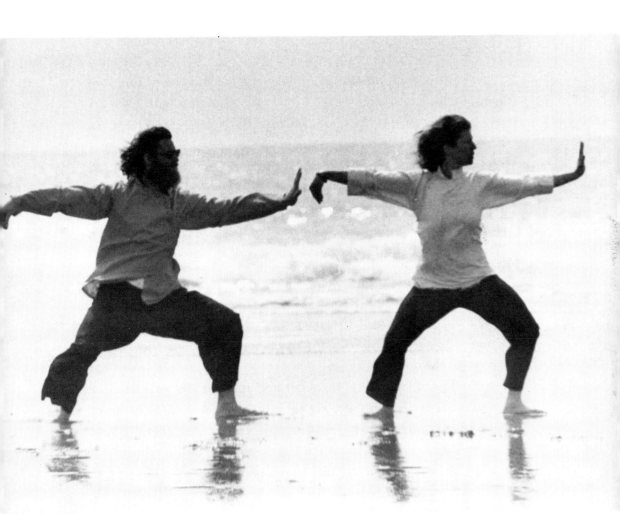

Empty Steps

In empty steps, all the body weight is on one foot. The foot without weight makes contact with the ground slightly, touching with either the heel or the toe. Both knees are bent. In Grasp the Swallow's Tail, paragraph 2b of the Form, we have the first-occurring empty step. All the body weight is on the left foot, while the right foot is beside it with no weight at all. The right foot is empty. There are several variations of the empty step, as in paragraph 1a, the left foot is empty; paragraph 6, the right foot, while empty, is in front, not beside the other foot.

The Hands

During performance the hands and arms are loose and engage in no physical exertion. In the open hand positions there is air between the fingers. When there is a fist, it is not clenched tightly. When punching, the wrist and forearm are in a straight line (the wrist is unbent). Force is not expelled. The Internal System concentrates on gathering chi (your vital energy), and developing inner power concealed in softness. The training is subtle and not obvious. It transcends mere physical training.

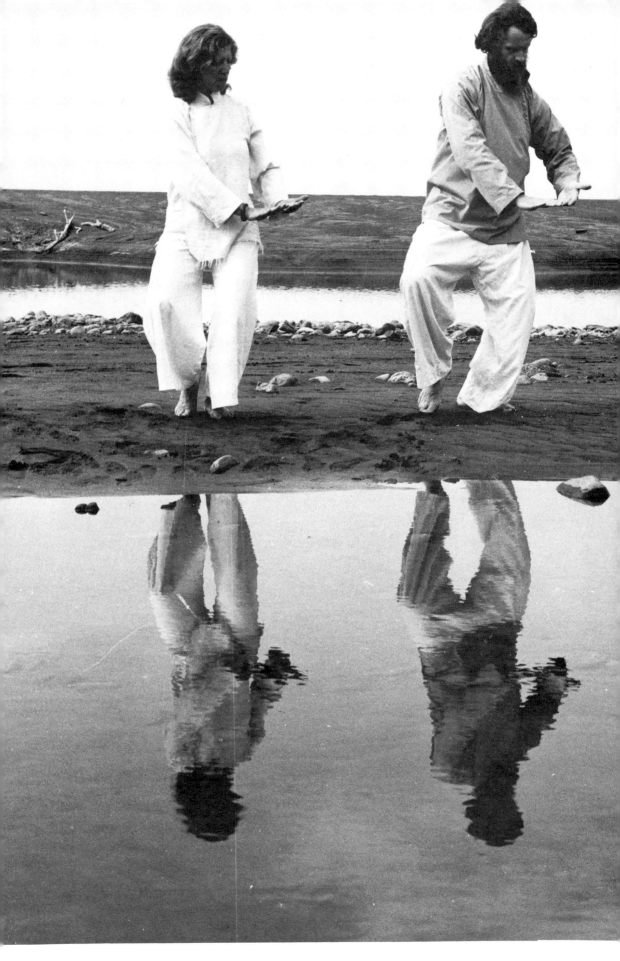

TAI CHI: THE FORM

How to Use This Manual

Here's the "How to Do It" portion of Kuang Ping Tai Chi. Imagine that you are the person in the picture. We recommend that during practice you start facing north with south behind. Enjoy trying it. Try to learn two or three movements when they are easy, and repeat them several times until you are ready to learn more. Linking the movements together without pause and keeping a consistent pace is the result of many repetitions and good concentration.

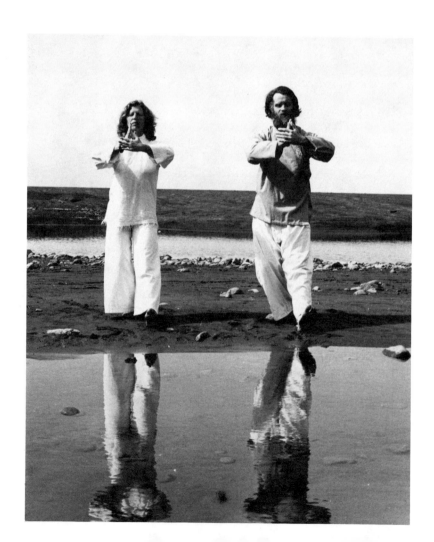

1. Homage to Buddha

Face north. Bend your knees and extend the left leg, bringing it to rest on its heel. All the body weight rests on the right foot. Raise your arms up to shoulder height and bring the hands together in the gesture of homage, as shown in the photo. This is an opening salute to the Divine in the universe, and within ourselves—our own Buddha nature.

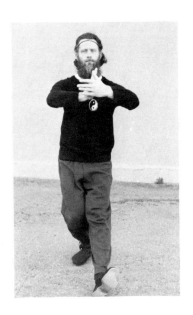

2. Grasp the Swallow's Tail (left side)

a. Step back and left with the left foot, shifting all the body weight onto it. Rest the right foot on its heel, toes pointing up. Both arms move in a downward arc to the left hip. The left elbow is angled. The left hand is palm up, and the right is palm down.

b. Step back with the right foot, bringing it beside the left in an empty step, touching the toes to the ground and raising the heel. See instructions for the empty step at the beginning of this section.

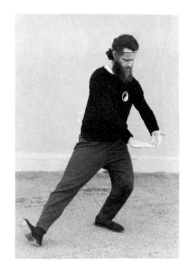

3. Press Forward and Push

Step northeast with the right foot into a T step, keeping both knees well bent. At the same time press forward and push with both hands, turning the waist so that the wrists are parallel and the palms are facing outward. At the conclusion of the push, the fingertips are level with the shoulders, hands are aligned above the right knee, and the waist has turned to the right in conformance with the hand movement. The center of balance is on the right leg.

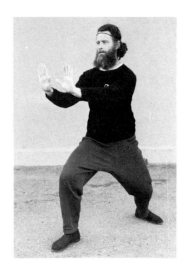

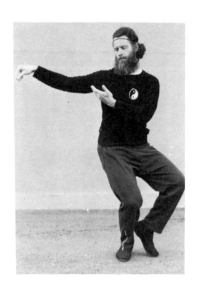

4. Step Up—Empty Step

a. Pivot to the north on the right heel. Bring the left foot forward next to it in an empty step.

b. Extend the right arm directly to the right, at shoulder height, and bend the hand down at the wrist. The thumb and index fingers touch each other. Keep the fingers bent. This is called a hooked hand or chicken's beak hand. This position for the right arm is retained throughout the next movement, Single Whip which follows. Bring the left arm in front of the chest; the palm is up and positioned under the right armpit, as shown.

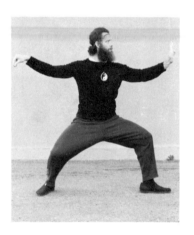

5. Single Whip

Step left, west, with the left foot, into a T step, placing the heel down first. Extend the left arm completely to the left and when it is fully extended, turn the palm out and push, at the same time sinking down into a lower, deeper stance, shifting the center of balance to the left leg. Keep your hips forward and flex the knees outward. The body faces north, arms are outstretched, elbows unbent, but not tense or rigid.

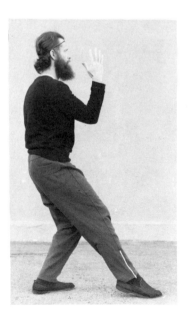

6. Stork Cools Its Wings

Keeping both knees bent and not moving the left foot, step left to the west with the right foot, turning the body and resting the right foot on its toe in an empty step; all the weight is now on the left foot and the body is facing west. At the same time, bring the right hooked hand forward and open it as if cutting or chopping, and the left hand to the left side, palm down, as shown in the photo.

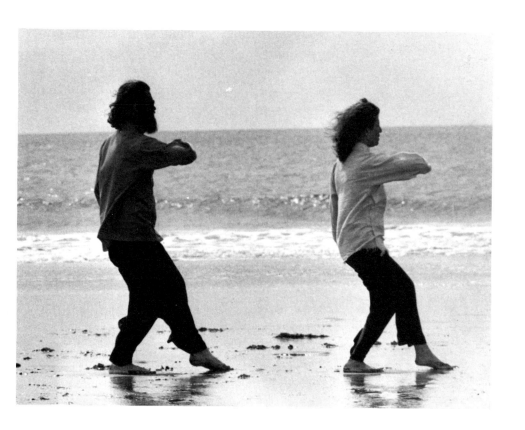

7. Elbow Strike

Step directly back and to the right with the right foot in a step shaped like the letter "L." At the same time as the leg movement, bring the right arm to a horizontal position at the chest. Now step back with the left leg in a reverse L step and bring it in front, resting on the toes.

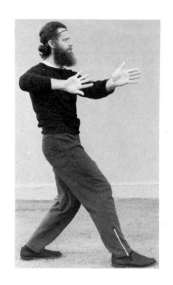 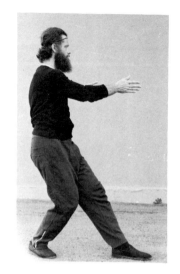 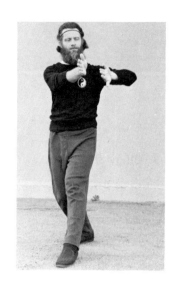

8. Deflect to the Side

a. Continuing the above, step directly back with the left foot, being careful not to turn it out. Raise both hands to shoulder height at the right side and push to the right as if deflecting a blow to the right side.

b. Step back with the right foot and push to the left side; the right hand is in front of the left.

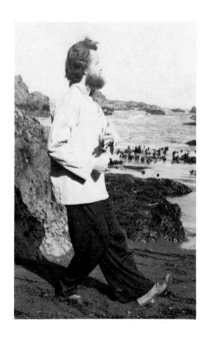

9. Deflect Downward

Bring the left hand forward with the palm toward you, and turn the right foot out 90 degrees; place all your weight on it, raising the left toe, keeping the heel down. Bring both hands down to the right hip with the left palm over the right wrist. The right hand now becomes a loosely held fist. This is a deflecting downward action, in front of and across the body.

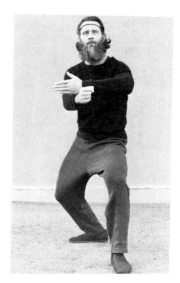

10. Parry and Punch

Punch in an upward arc with the right hand, to shoulder height and toward the center line of the body. The left hand guards the right and pushes upward at the same time as the punch. Bend the knees deeply and shift about 60 percent of the body weight to the left foot, which is now firmly placed. Your right foot is turned out 90 degrees. Hold the fist loosely but tighten it momentarily at the conclusion of the punch, using only slightly more energy. Twist the waist and right hip into the punch. The arms are not tensed at the end of the punch. The elbows are loose.

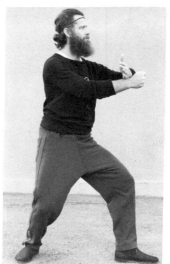

11. Divide Upward, Guard the Temples

Draw the hands back to the temples, shifting all the weight to the right leg and pointing the toes upward.

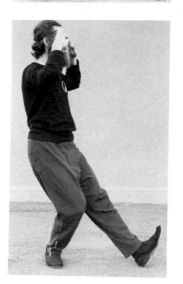

55

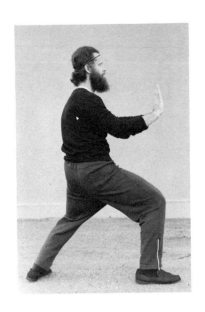

12. Step Forward, Push

Pivot on the left heel, turning the foot outward 90 degrees. Step forward with the right foot into a T stance and push forward with both hands. The fingertips are at shoulder height and the wrists are parallel during the push. At the conclusion of the push the hands will center over the right knee. You are facing west. The center of balance is the right leg.

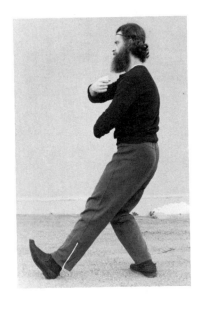

13. Counter-Clockwise Turn and Carry Tiger to Mountain

Pivot completely around 180 degrees to the east. First pivot 90 degrees on the right heel. The right foot now points to the south. Pivot on the left heel, with the toe pointing up, so that the left foot now points east. At the same time, your body turns to the left. The arms move in front of the body with the right vertical fist placed over the left elbow. The left open palm is facing you, and under the right elbow. The hands are held as though carrying a rectangular box.

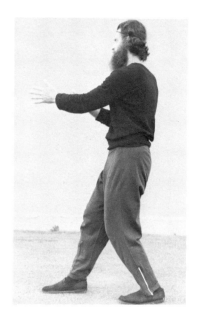

14. Walk Forward, Both Hands Circularly Blocking

Extend the hands in front of the chest so that the right fingertips almost touch the left wrist. The following movements are a series of circles performed at a ratio of one-half circle to one step. Take a step forward with the left foot and circle both hands clockwise toward the left half of the circle; step again, with the right foot, and continue the circle to the right. Step again with the left and continue the circle from right to left. Step once more with the right foot and continue the hand circling toward the right side. This same circling technique can be seen in Western and Chinese fencing and is used to screen out or intercept all body attacks.

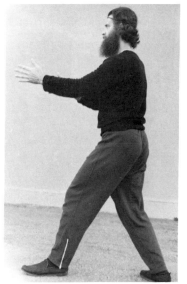

15. Step Forward, Parry, and Punch

From the above position, turn the right foot outward on the heel 90 degrees, step forward into a T with the left foot forward, placing about 60 percent of the body weight on it. Punch in an arc with the right vertical fist, guarding it at the wrist with the left hand. This is a short punch.

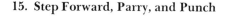

57

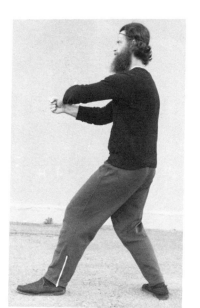

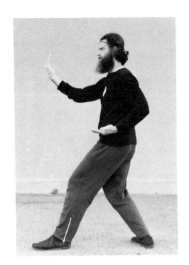
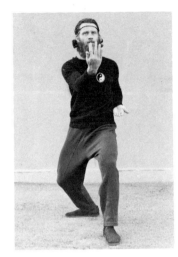

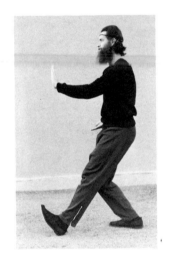

16. Backhand Slap

Open the right hand and bring it over the left in an open hand slap. At the same time bring the left hand near the left hip with the hand open and palm up. After the slap the right continues in a downward arc to the hip with the palm down. The left hand rises to shoulder level and pushes out directly in front of the body with the palm facing outward, its fingers pointing up. As you push, rest your left foot on the heel, toes up. All the weight is now on the right leg.

17. Repulse the Monkey, Three Retreating Steps

a. Step back with the left foot, placing the toe down first. It is turned out 45 degrees. Bring the left hand down to the left hip, palm up. At the same time lift the right hand to the height of the armpit, with the palm up. Extend the right arm straight to the front in a pushing action. The right leg is extended and on its heel, toes pointing up. This is a retreating step. Repeat it twice more as described.

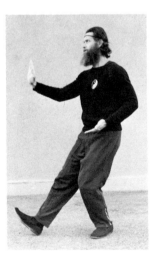

b. Step back with the right foot, turning it out 45 degrees and lower the right hand in a descend-

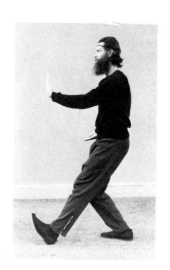

ing arc to the right hip. Raise the left hand to the height of the armpit, palm turned out, and push. The left leg is now extended, heel down, toes up.

c. For the third step, repeat the procedure in 17a.

18. Side Pivot, Cross Wrists

Pivot the left foot on its heel 90 degrees so that it faces northwest and bring the right foot back on the toe close to the left, in an empty step. Move the hands slowly downward and position them in front of the groin, wrists crossed, left hand over right; the left palm faces the body, the right palm faces outward.

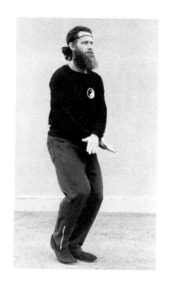

19. White Crane Flying

Step out in a wide T stance with the toe of the right foot pointed to the northeast. While stepping, spread both arms wide. The arms look like a bird's wings with the right arm extended to a height of three inches above the shoulder; the left hand aligns with the waist. Both palms are back.

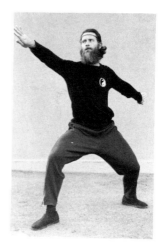

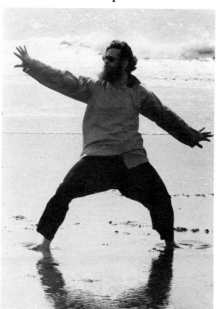

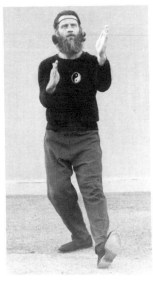

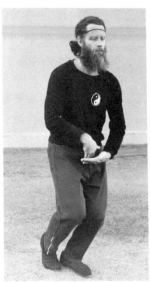

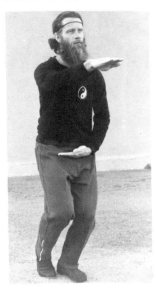

20. Raise Left Hand, Raise Right Hand

a. You are facing north. Step forward with the left foot onto the left heel, toes up, bringing both hands to the front, with the palms facing each other. The fingertips of the right hand are level with the wrist of the left hand. The elbows are close to the body.

b. Step forward again with the left foot, bringing the right foot forward next to the left in an empty step.

c. While the foot action is occurring, the left hand moves to the abdomen, palm up. Move the right hand down, fingertips over the left hand, and sweep the left palm, as if brushing away dust. Extend the right hand straight forward to shoulder height. Step back with the right foot and bring the right hand back to where it was for the opening position of the posture. Raise up the left toes. Keep the right elbow bent and raise it to shoulder height, palm down.

21. Turn Directly Around and Raise the Right Hand, Then the Left

a. Turn completely around clockwise, pivoting on the left heel to the southeast, putting all your weight on the left foot and coming to rest with the right foot on its heel. No step has been taken. As you pivot, raise the right elbow to shoulder height and at the end of the pivot, lower it again to its original position. You are now facing south. Move your arms directly in front of the body with the palms facing each other. Bring the right hand forward and the left fingertips align with the right wrist. The elbows are close to the body.

b. Step forward with the right foot and bring the

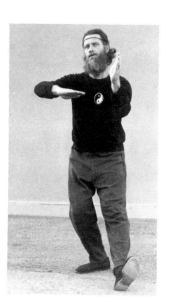
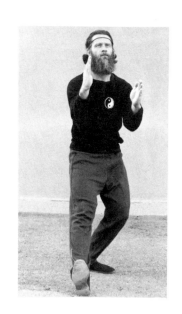
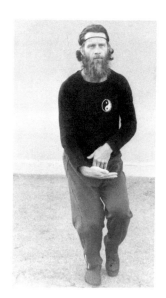

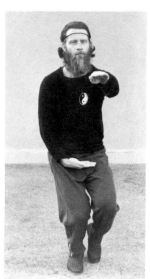

left foot forward next to the right in an empty
step.
c. While the foot action is occurring, the right
hand drops to the abdomen, palm up. The left
hand moves down, fingertips over the right hand,
and sweeps the right hand as if brushing away
dust. Step back with the left foot and extend the
left hand forward as in the opening position,
21a.

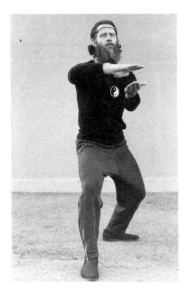

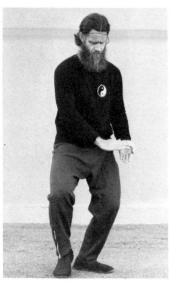

22. Grab and Pull Back

a. Extend the arms and reach out as if grabbing someone's arm or fist. When reaching forward, place the right foot flat on the ground with approximately 60 percent of the body weight shifting to the right leg.

b. Now pull back, moving both hands downward to the left hip. Also return the right foot close to the left in an empty step.

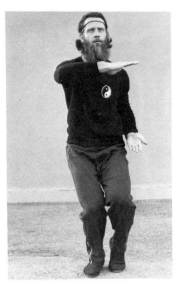

23. Step Up and Open Hand Strike

Still facing south, step forward with your right foot, bringing the left foot forward next to the right in an empty step. While doing so, raise your right arm, bent at the elbow, to shoulder height. The right foot and the right arm move in unison. The left hand does not move.

24. Draw the Bow

Step left, east, with the left foot into a T stance. The right hand moves to the temple, while the left arm extends fully to the left and the head turns left so that the gaze is on the left hand. Sink the body weight down as far as it will go by flexing the knees more deeply, while keeping the hips forward.

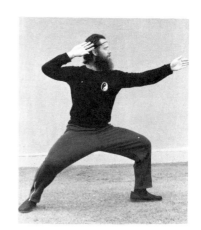

25. Green Dragon Step

a. Pivot the left foot on the heel 45 degrees to the right. Take a small step forward with the right foot. Reach out to the right with both hands. The arms and hands are positioned at shoulder height with the hands facing inward toward each other. The right hand is in front and the elbows are close to the body.

b. Now reach both hands forward and pull them back, bringing them to the waist and returning the right foot to the left in an empty step. All the weight is on the left foot.

c. Next, step forward to the southwest with the right foot first, following with the left foot in an empty step. Push both arms upward to the southwest, palms facing away from you. Keep the hands together. Imagine you are offbalancing an opponent.

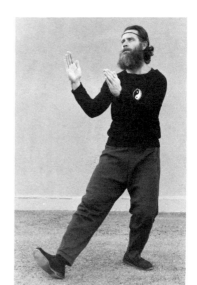

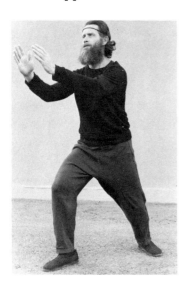

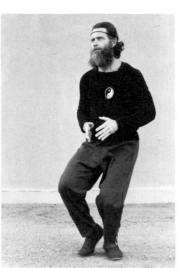

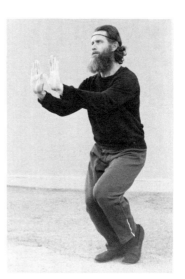

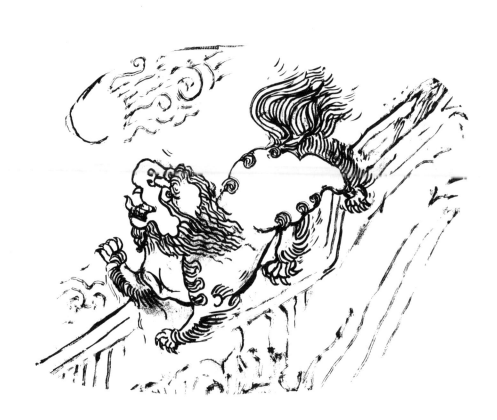

26. Single Whip

Pivot the right foot 45 degrees left, and step left into the Single Whip position. Follow the general instructions for paragraph 5. The left hand now faces east. The body faces south.

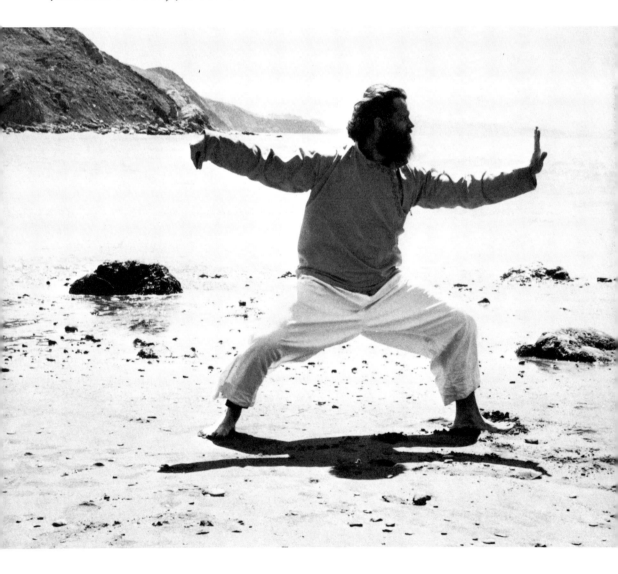

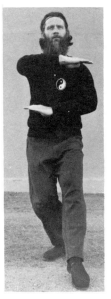

27. Transition Step for Wave Hands Like Clouds

Bring the left foot forward onto its toes in an empty step. Move your arms in front of the body. The right hand is shoulder height, while the left hand is under the right elbow. Both palms face down.

28. Wave Hands Like Clouds

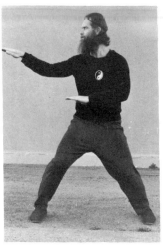

a. You are still facing south but proceeding to the east. Step left, placing the entire foot down at the same time (flat-footed, not heel first or toe first). Both feet are now parallel. Extend the right arm to the right, palm down.

b. Now the left hand rises to the height of the chest, and the right foot joins the left. The movement is completed when the left arm (which was in front of the chest) is fully extended to the left side of the body at shoulder height while the right hand is lowered to your navel.

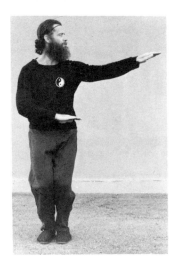

c. Repeat paragraphs 28a and b. Now assume the hand position preceding Single Whip, 4b. The right hand extends fully to the side in a hooked, or chicken's beak, hand. The left hand is in front of the chest, next to the right armpit and close to the body, with the palm up. The left foot is in the empty step and all the body's weight is on the right foot.

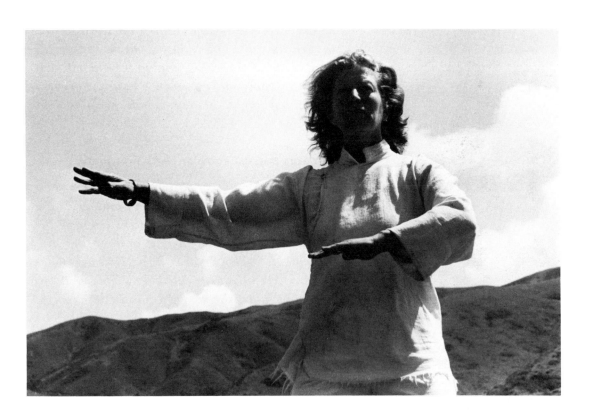

29. Single Whip

Repeat paragraph 5 for hand and foot movements. There is no directional change, here. You are still facing south. The left hand points east.

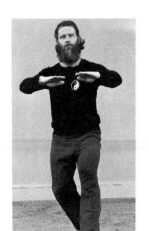

30. Pat the Horse

Retract the left leg about one foot length onto its toe in an empty step, shifting the waist to face toward the east. The right leg has all the weight on it. Extend the arms, keeping the elbows bent and the palms facing down. The arms form a circle; the fingers of both hands point toward each other.

31. Step Forward and Circular Block Downward

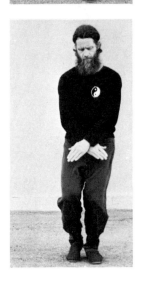

Step forward with the left foot bringing the right foot beside it in an empty step, and drop the hands down, crossing the wrists in front of the groin; palms face the body. Continue the arm movement, sweeping in a large circular movement overhead and to the sides. This is a circular block. All the weight is on the left foot.

32. Side Heel Thrust Kicks, Right and Left

In performing these kicks, paragraphs 32 and 33, thrust with the heel, and point the toe up.

a. Continuing the above, when the right hand is at shoulder height, extend the right leg completely to the right side. Then both arms and the right leg descend together.

b. And continuing without stopping the action, there are again crossed wrists, palms in at the groin, and a large sweeping circular block overhead, with the left leg completely extended to the left side, while the arms descend as the leg descends.

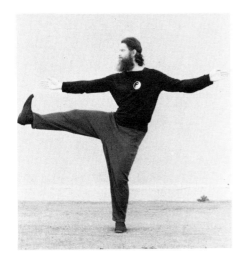
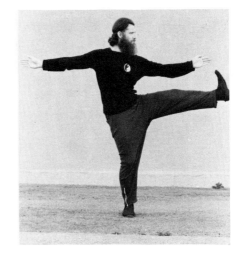

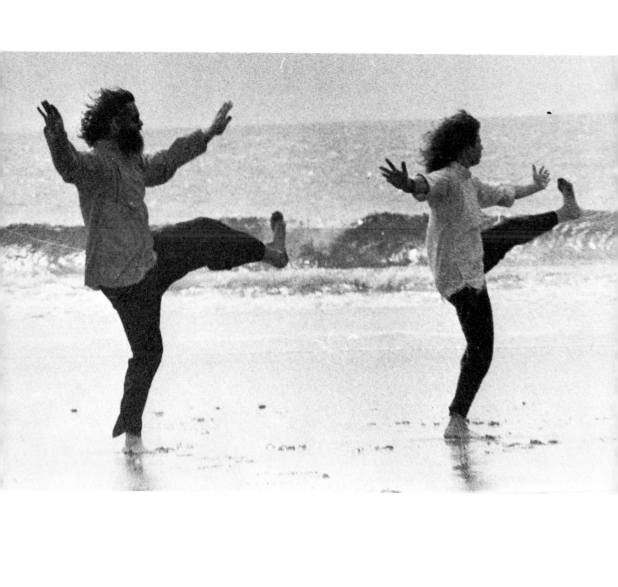

33. Diagonal Turn and Left Thrust Kick

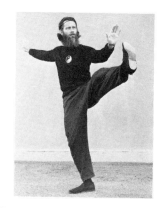

When bringing the left foot down in the preceding paragraph, place it in an empty step on the toe, behind the heel of the right foot. Pivot left 135 degrees on the right heel, to the northwest, turning the body diagonally to the left. Perform the circular block again and kick again with the left leg.

34. Wind Blowing the Lotus Leaf

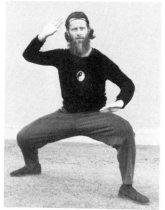

a. When bringing the left foot down in the above kick, bring it down into a T step, with the left toe facing southwest. Your right hand comes up to the right temple, palm facing outward. The left hand is palm downward and is positioned on the inside of the left knee.

b. Pivot the left foot out 90 degrees to the southeast and step to the southwest with the right foot, shifting the body's weight to the left foot, and coming to rest in a T stance again. While the foot action goes on, the arms move as follows: Sweep the left palm backward and then block upward in a circular motion at the side of the body and place it in front of the left temple, palm facing outward. The right arm comes to rest above the inside of the right knee, palm down.

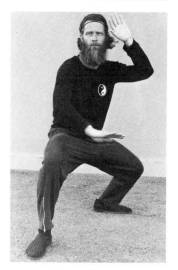

c. Continuing this movement, pivot the right foot out to the northwest 90 degrees and turn the body completely around 180 degrees, stepping southwest with the left foot. The arms move again as described above: Sweep the right hand backward from the right knee, and then block upward in a circular motion, coming to rest in front of the right temple, palm facing out. Move the left hand from beside the left temple to the inside of the left knee, with the palm down. You are now in a T stance.

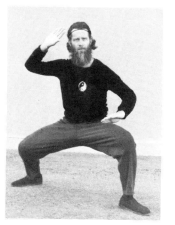

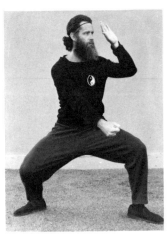

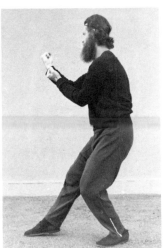

35. Open Palm Upward Block, with Diagonal Punch Down

Sweep the left knee in a circular block with the left hand and bring it to the left temple, palm out. Punch downward diagonally toward your left knee with the right vertical fist.

36. Pivot Around, Forearm Block

Turn the body without taking a step by pivoting on the left heel (it becomes the back leg) 135 degrees to the right and turning your right foot so that the toes point northeast. The hands both block in an upward arc and come to rest with the right fist pointed northeast and at the height of your eyes. The left fist is parallel to the right, and it aligns with the wrist of the right hand. For self-defense, the movement can be used as a back knuckle strike or a forearm block.

37. Flying Jump Kick

a. Step northeast with the right foot and simultaneously raise the left knee high, jumping into the air and kicking straight outward with the right toe. As the left foot returns to the ground, chop downward with the left fist while making a circle downward, and open the right palm, slapping the right instep with it as you kick out your right foot.
b. You land on the left foot, still facing northeast.

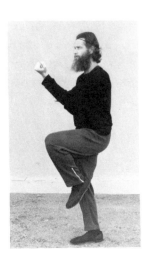

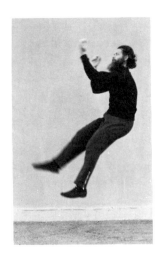

38. Step In, Deflect Downward, Parry, and Punch

Step northeast with the right foot into a T stance. Bring the left foot forward. Parry by extending the left arm across the front of the body to the middle of the chest. Punch forward with the right vertical fist and place it under the left wrist.

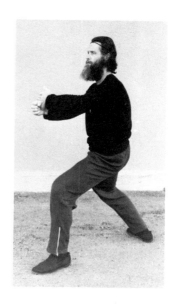

39. Step Back, Sweep with the Wrists

a. Following the conclusion of the above punch, place all weight on the left foot. Step back directly with the right, transferring all the weight to it.

b. The left foot is extended in front of the body in an empty step. Move both arms in a downward arc to the sides of the body. Bend the wrists; palms face downward.

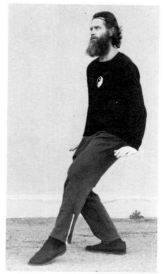

73

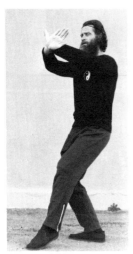
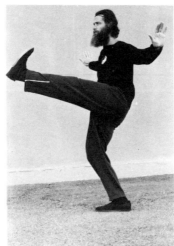
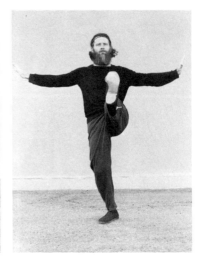

40. Circular Block and Kick with the Left Heel

Cross both wrists in front of the groin, palms in, and continue the arm movement in a circular block up in front of the face and out to the sides. When the arms are overhead, and as they descend, kick out to the northeast with the left foot, fully extending the heel and pointing the toe toward your face. This is a slow leg raise and is performed in the slow pace of Tai Chi, not abruptly.

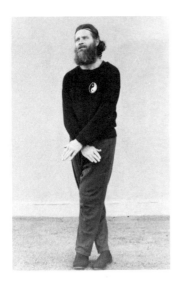

41. Heel Swivel, Cross Wrists, and Pivot Around

Continuing the movement of the left foot, bring it down on the heel and place it behind the heel of the right foot. The hands descend and cross at the wrists in front of the groin. Turn completely around by rising on the toe of the right foot and the heel of the left. The body is now facing northwest.

42. Circular Block and Right Heel Kick

Now raise the arms in a circular block upward and kick with the right heel extended to the northeast.

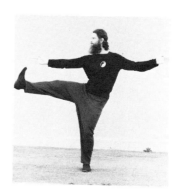

43. Step In, Parry, and Punch

After you lower the right kicking leg, step onto it, into a T stance by bringing the left foot forward. Punch forward with the right vertical fist and bring it under the wrist of the left hand. The left arm is guarding the body. You are now facing northeast.

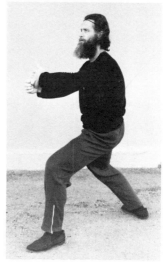

44. Close Up, Guard the Temples

Still facing northeast, roll back, putting all the weight on the right leg, momentarily raising the toe of the left foot, keeping the heel down. Raise your hands to the temples, keeping the elbows bent.

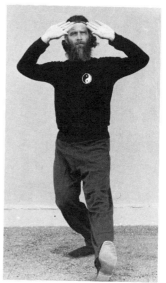

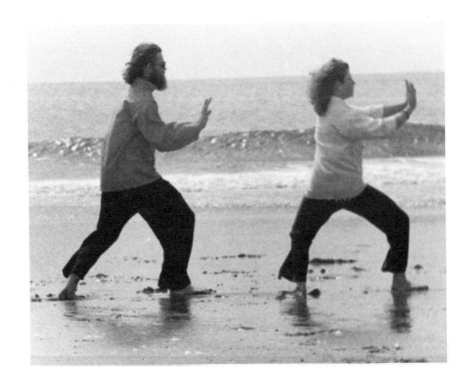

45. **Press Forward and Push**

Shift 60 percent of your weight onto the left foot and press forward with both hands fully extended, wrists bent, palms facing out, and fingertips pointed upward at shoulder height.

46. **Reverse T Step**

Move the left hand palm down over the right wrist. The right hand is held in an upturned fist. Both hands are chest height. Place your left foot in front of the right, with the left instep facing the right toe.

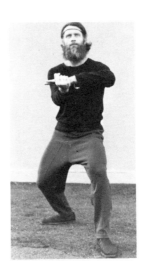
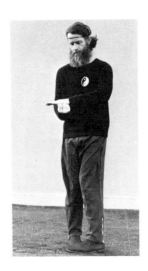

47. Elbow Chop

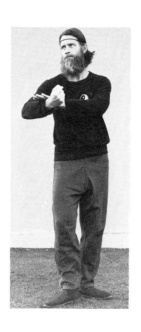

Turn your body to the northwest and point the right toe in that same direction. All the weight is on the left foot. Take a wide step with the right foot to the northwest, bringing the left foot behind the heel of the right foot in a closed T step. While taking this step, both arms move to the right of the body, chopping upward. The left hand is palm down, over the upturned right fist.

48. Retreat Downward

Step left with the left foot and turn the right foot 90 degrees to the left so that it is parallel with the left foot. Bend the left knee and bring the body down squatting to the left (as in the warmup, Tiger Crouches Downward). The arms descend to chest height, moving left with the body; the right fist turns over, palm down, and remains under the open left hand.

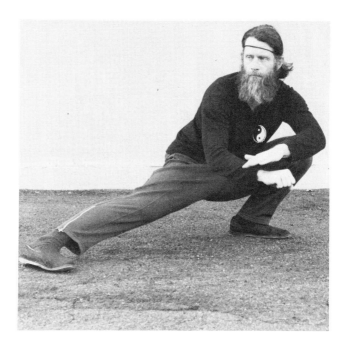

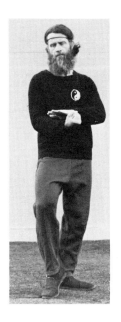 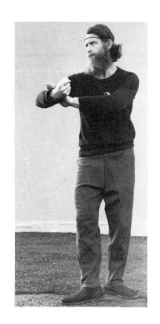

49. Rise Up and Chop Again

Rise to standing position, bringing the left leg next to the right in an empty step, and bring both arms to the right of the body in an Elbow Chop, as described in paragraph 47. When you chop upward, the right fist is again palm up, as in paragraph 47.

50. Diagonal Single Whip

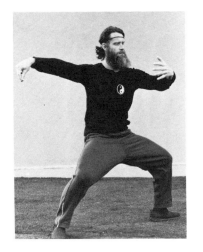

Step left, to the southeast, with the left foot, keeping the toe pointed toward the southeast. Perform the Single Whip movement as described in paragraphs 4 and 5. Turn the body so that you are progressing diagonally from the northwest to southeast. The Diagonal Single Whip is a variation of the Single Whip hand and arm movement. The left hand, which is usually palm up at the beginning of Single Whip now faces the body. The elbow should be at shoulder level at the completion of the step.

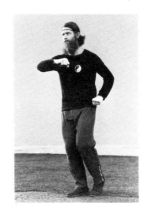

51. Wild Horse Flinging Its Mane

a. Draw the left foot back to the right in an empty step. Turn the torso so you face south. Both hands become loose fists. At the same time bring the left fist down to the left hip. It comes to rest beside the left hip. Move the right arm in toward the body, at the chest.

b. Step diagonally left with the left foot, toward the southeast, and place the right foot in an empty step beside the left. Punch toward the right with the right fist in a downward arc to rest beside the right hip. At the same time, raise the left fist up to shoulder height. This is the first step of a two-step sequence.

c. Now step diagonally right with the right foot toward the southwest and place the left foot in an empty step beside the right. Punch downward to the left with the left hand and raise the right to shoulder height.

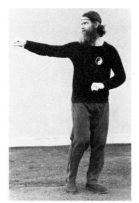

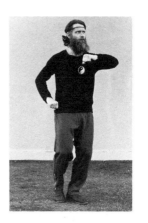

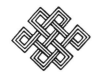

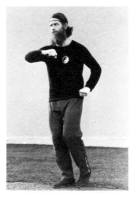

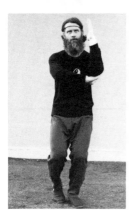

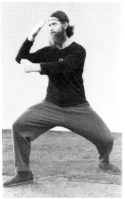

52. Diagonal Single Whip

Now bring the right hand to the right side forming the chicken's beak hand, a hooked hand; and the left palm facing in toward the chest as described in paragraph 50. This is the same as in paragraph 50. The Diagonal Single Whip is done to the southeast. Illustrated on page 78.

53. Fair Lady Working at the Loom (Steps in Four Directions)

a. Turn the left foot 45 degrees to the south and bring the toe of the right foot beside the heel of the left foot, resting in an empty step. Bring the right hand under the left elbow as illustrated. You are now facing south.

b. Turn completely around by pivoting on the left heel and right toe. After turning, continue the movement by taking a wide step with the right foot to the northeast into a T stance. Keep the knees well bent and take wide steps throughout these postures. Draw the left arm to the left side, forearm facing up, and make a fist. Bring the right hand in an open-palm upward block to the right temple. Complete Fair Lady Working at the Loom by punching with the left fist and turning the waist to the right while punching. You are punching toward the northeast. At the last moment twist the fist so that it is vertical and facing the right forearm. This is the first step.

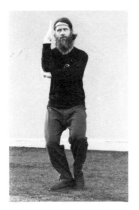

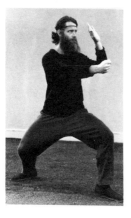

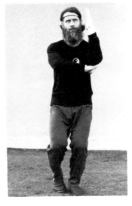

c. Step forward in an empty step with the left foot, bringing it next to the right. At the same time, bring the left open palm under the right elbow, with the right arm pointing up and the hand open. This is a transitional step.

d. Step left with the left foot to the northwest into a T stance. Draw the right arm to the right side, forearm facing up; the hand is a closed fist. Bring the left hand in an open-palm upward block to the left temple. Complete the above by punching with the right fist, turning it vertically. Turn the torso to the left in the direction of the punch, which is northwest. Extend the arm completely at shoulder level. This is the second direction.

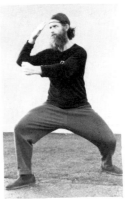

e. Proceeding to the third direction, turn the left foot 45 degrees to point north and bring the right foot behind the left heel. Hands and feet as in paragraph 53a. Turn completely around by pivoting on the left heel.

f. Continue the movement by taking a wide step with the right foot, to the southwest, into a T stance. Draw the left arm to the left side, making a fist. Execute an open-palm upward block to the right temple, as you punch with the left vertical fist. This completes the third direction.

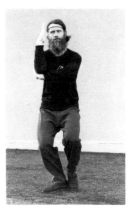

g. Step forward in an empty step with the left foot, bringing it next to the right. At the same time, bring the left open palm under the right elbow, with the right arm pointing up and the hand open.

h. Proceeding to the fourth direction, step to the southeast with the left foot, into a T stance. Draw the right arm to the right side making a fist as in 53d. Block up with the open left palm to the temple as you punch with the right fist.

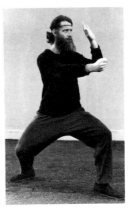

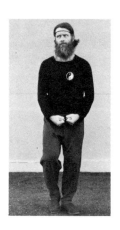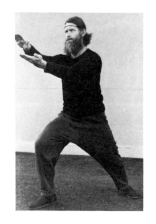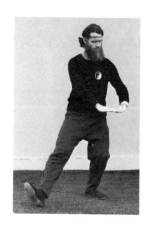

54. Grasp the Swallow's Tail (Variant)

a. Bring the right foot forward beside the left in an empty step. Drop the hands in front of the groin. Both hands are loose fists facing inward.

b. Step to the right with the right foot pointing southwest. Reach in front of your chest with both hands; the left is under the right and palm up; the right is palm down.

c. Next, both arms move downward in an arc to the left hip with the left elbow angled out. Raise the right foot onto the heel; toes are up. The movement simulates grasping an opponent's arm, pulling it down and back, and, when he resists, pushing him forward. This is basically the same form as in paragraph 2, with slight variation in the footwork.

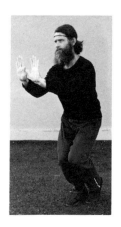

55. Push Forward

Next, step forward and push, bringing the left leg forward, beside the right into an empty step. The push is the same as in paragraph 3, except that this time you have stepped forward. Keep your palms together when pushing, with the fingertips chest height. You are pushing an imaginary opponent backward and upward. The push is to the southwest. You are again in T stance.

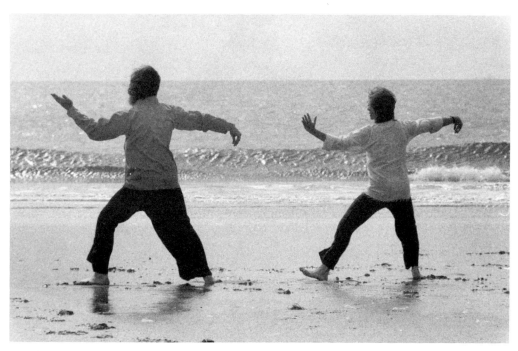

56. Single Whip

There's a small adjustment step now. Pivot the right foot, now facing southwest, 45 degrees, to the south. Repeat movements for Single Whip as in paragraph 5. The left hand pushes to the east.

57. Wave Hands Like Clouds

Repeat instructions for paragraphs 27 and 28.

58. Single Whip

Repeat movements for Single Whip as in paragraph 5. You are still facing south. The Single Whip movement is to the east.

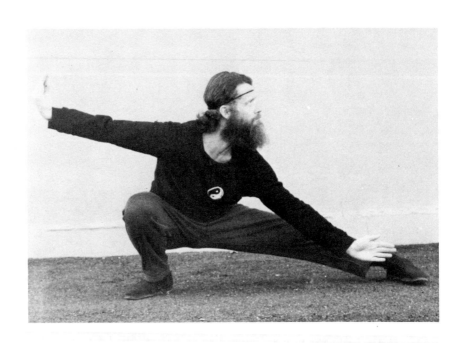

59. Snake Creeps Down

From the Single Whip posture, pivot the left foot, now pointing east, 90 degrees to point south. Bend the right knee deeply and bring the whole body down, squatting to the right. The left leg is straight. In this position, keep your feet parallel and heels flat on the ground. Move the extended left hand from the left side of the body straight down to the left ankle. Raise your right arm above the shoulder and turn the right hand (chicken's beak hand) over in a counter-clockwise circle so that the wrist is facing the earth, and the fingers are pointing upward.

84

60. Golden Cock Stands on One Leg

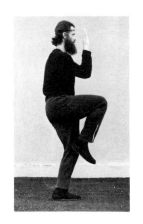

Pivot the left heel 90 degrees, and rise up on the left leg. You are facing east. Raise the right leg and bend your knee. Brush the thigh with the right open palm, pushing the arm forward in an arc extending in front of the body. Simultaneously, kick straight forward with a slow heel-thrusting kick. The left hand has remained at rest, palm facing backward at your left hip. Now lower the right foot and step forward. Raise the left knee up and brush the left thigh with the left open palm. Slowly kick straight forward with the left leg and push forward in an arc with the left hand. Bring the extended left leg directly down, resting on the heel with the toes up. At the conclusion of this position, the left hand is extended, and the right hand is at the right side, palm open, facing east. All the weight is on the back leg, the right. These steps may be repeated twice or four times.

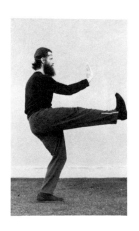

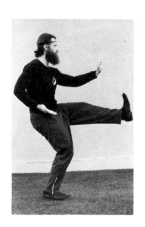

For movements 61 through 68, repeat movements as described in paragraphs 17 through 24. The compass directions for these movements are the same as before.

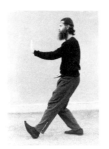 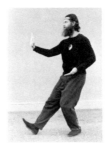 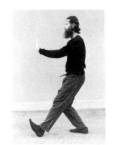

61. Repulse the Monkey

Repeat movements for paragraph 17. There are three retreating steps.

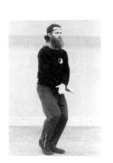

62. Side Pivot, Cross Wrists

Repeat movements for paragraph 18.

63. White Crane Flying

Repeat movements for paragraph 19.

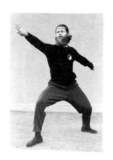

64. Raise Left Hand, Raise Right Hand

Follow instructions for paragraph 20 a, b, and c.

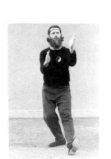 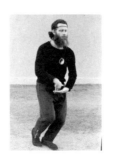 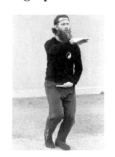

65. **Turn Directly Around and Raise Right Hand, Then Left Hand**

 Repeat paragraph 21 a, b, and c.

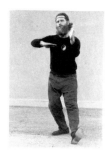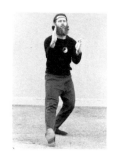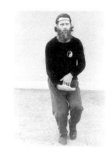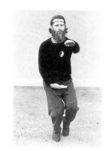

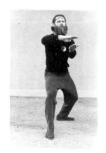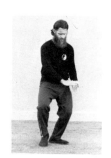

66. **Grab and Pull Back**

 Repeat paragraph 22.

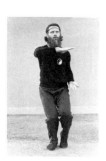

67. **Step Up and Open Hand Strike**

 Repeat movements for paragraph 23.

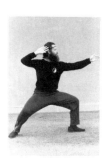

68. **Draw the Bow**

 Repeat movements for paragraph 24. You are in T stance gazing east at your extended left hand.

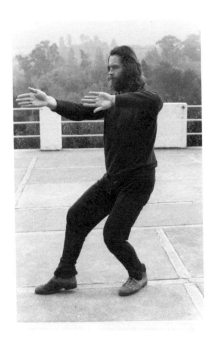

69. Deflect to the Side

Turn left by taking a step east with the right foot, bringing it well in front of the left in an empty step. All the weight is on the left foot (which has now become the back leg). Raise both arms to the left side, level with the left shoulder.

70. Push and Step

Step forward again to the east with the right foot and bring the left behind and close to the right. Push forward while stepping. Keep the fingertips level with the shoulders. Fingers point up, the wrists are bent, and the palms face outward, away from the body. When stepping keep the feet as close to and parallel with the ground as possible.

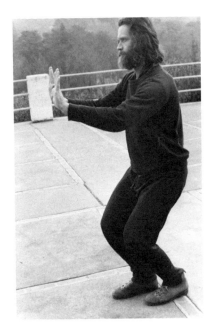

71. Strike Opponent's Ears

Step forward again, east, with the right foot, repeating the same step as in paragraph 70. At the same time, punch with both fists in a small semicircle. The fists are held horizontally. You are striking an opponent's temples or ears with the first two knuckles in a circular punch.

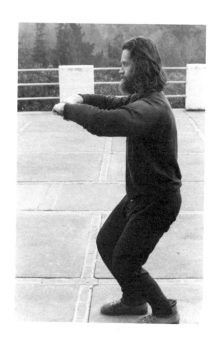

72. Cannon Fires Through the Sky

Step forward once more repeating same steps as in paragraphs 70 and 71. Punch in an upward diagonal arc with both fists; wrists and fists face upward. At the conclusion of this punch the right fist is extended beyond the left fist.

73. Single Whip

Turn the right foot north 90 degrees and step with the left foot into T stance, performing Single Whip to the west. Instructions for performance are the same as single whip in paragraph 5.

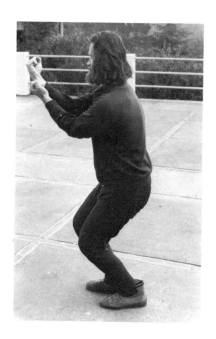

74. Wave Hands Like Clouds

Repeat the movements for paragraphs 27 and 28. Your body is facing north, but you are stepping toward the west.

75. Single Whip

Step with the left foot into T stance and perform Single Whip to the west, as before, in paragraph 73.

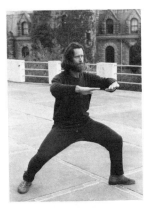

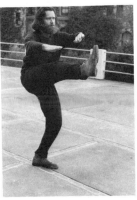

76. Water Lily Kick

a. Draw the weight back onto the right leg into the position of Pat the Horse, paragraph 30. Turn the right leg 45 degrees so that the toe points northwest.

b. Step left with the left foot to the southwest. Place all the weight on the left foot and kick with the right, raising it up in a sweeping, circular, clockwise motion. The toe is pointed in the direction of the kick. Brush the heel and toe of the right foot with your hands before the foot descends. When the kick is finished, you return your right foot to its starting position in T stance.

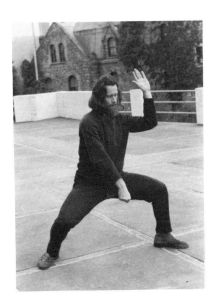

77. Punch Downward

The hands are still in front with the palms facing down as in Pat the Horse. Bring the left hand to the left temple and punch straight down with the right fist. As you punch, sink your weight downward by expanding the knees outward and deepening your T stance.

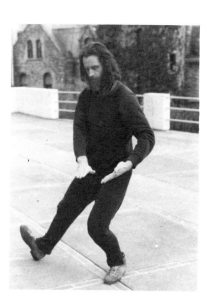

78. Step Up and Grasp the Swallow's Tail (Variant)

   Repeat paragraph 54.

79. Push Forward

   Repeat paragraph 55.

80. Single Whip

   Repeat paragraph 56. You are facing south; the left palm points east.

81. Wave Hands Like Clouds

   Repeat paragraphs 27 and 28 a and b. There is no directional change.

82. Single Whip

   Repeat movements for paragraph 80. The left hand pushes east.

83. Snake Creeps Down

   Repeat paragraph 59.

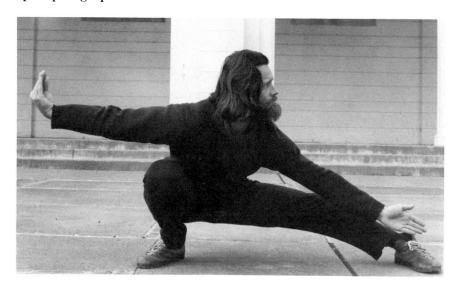

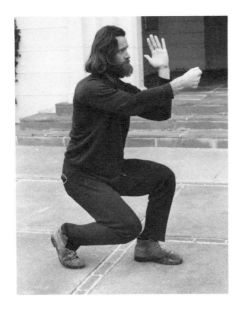

84. Seven Star Punch

Turn the left foot out so the toes face east. Bring the right foot forward beside the left in an empty step. Bend the knees very deeply and remain in a low body posture. Punch forward with the right hand from the side of the chest with the fist vertical. Bend the left arm at the elbow. The left open palm faces the right fist and guards it.

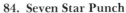

85. Retreat and Ride the Tiger

Step back with the right foot and turn the toe south so that you are in a T stance. Extend the left hand in the Single Whip hand position. The right hand is held in the chicken's beak position in back of the body at shoulder height, wrist turned downward, fingers pointing up as in paragraph 59.

86. Slant the Body and Turn the Moon

a. Step south with the left toe (empty step) and place all the weight on the back foot (right), which now pivots 45 degrees to the southwest. You are turned to the south. Move the right hand to the left, keeping it at shoulder level. Move your left arm behind the body; the hand is in a chicken's beak, fingers turned up. Look to the rear, over your left shoulder, before performing the next movement.

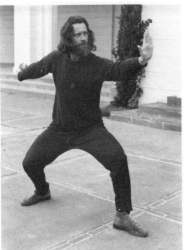
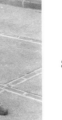

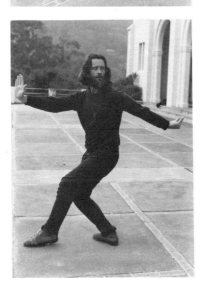

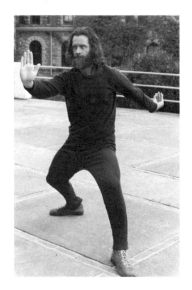

b. Pivot on the right heel, turning the body 180 degrees to the right. Take a large circular step with the left foot and place it down facing northwest. You are now in the T stance. The hands have not moved from their position in paragraph 86a.

87. Water Lily Kick

Bring the arms forward, as in Pat the Horse. Kick with the right foot in a sweeping, clockwise, circular motion, brushing the down-turned hands with the instep of the right foot. When the kick is completed, return the right foot to a T stance. See paragraph 76. The kick can be used as a reverse roundhouse or leg sweep; in Pat the Horse you are grasping an opponent's arm.

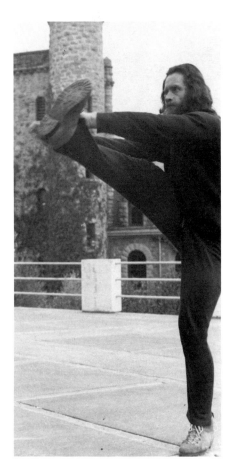

93

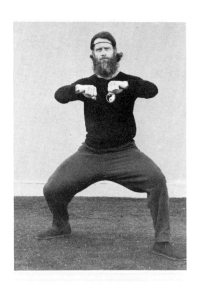

L. R.

88. Shoot the Tiger

Next, punch in circles by moving the right hand in counter-clockwise spirals and the left hand in clockwise spirals, as in the diagram. The punches are performed on a horizontal plane, as if polishing a table top. Punch six times in small, spiraling movements, first with the right hand as the left draws back and then with the left as the right draws back.

89. Grasp the Swallow's Tail

Step forward into empty step and then, to the right with the right foot into T stance facing northeast. Reach the arms out to the right, northeast, at shoulder height. Next, pull back, bringing the arms down to the left hip. The right palm faces down, the left up. All the body weight is transferred to the left foot when pulling back the hands. The right foot is resting on the heel, toes pointing up.

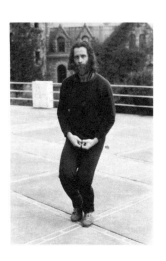

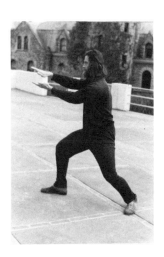

94

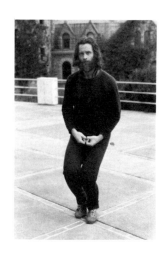

90. Push Forward

The arms push forward to the right, while the right foot is placed flat on the ground and the body is in T stance. See also paragraph 3.

91. Step Back

Bring the right foot back to the left in an empty step and drop the hands down into fists in front of the groin.

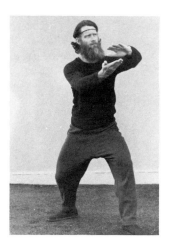

92. Grasp the Swallow's Tail

Step back and southeast, to the right, with the right foot. Reach the hands to the left, the left palm facing downward and the right facing up. Next, pull both hands back toward the right hip; the left open palm faces down, and the right open palm faces up. Bring the left foot onto its heel, toes pointing up.

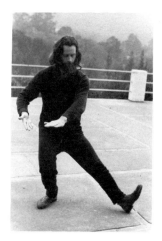

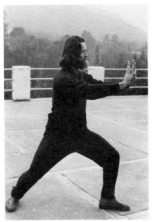

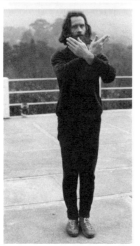

93. Push Forward

The arms push forward to the left, while the left foot is placed flat on the ground and the body is in T stance.

94. Cross Hands and Circle Overhead

Step back with the left foot, bringing it beside the right. Cross the wrists in front of the chest, left over right, palms toward the chest, arms in a circle in front of the body. Continue moving the hands very slowly downward to the sides of the body and then reaching overhead, bending at the elbows and slowly returning the hands down to a natural standing position. This is the closing posture of Tai Chi Chuan.

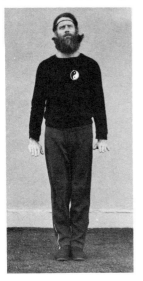

96

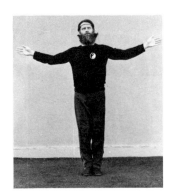

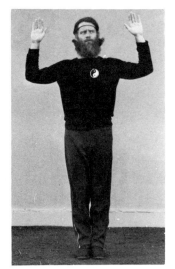

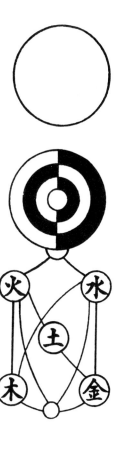

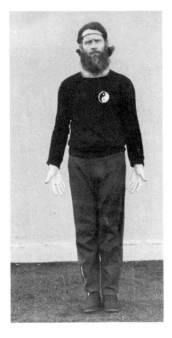

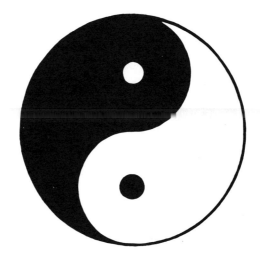

From the I Ching

The Creative manifests itself in the head, the Receptive in the belly, the Arousing in the foot, the Gentle in the thighs, the Abysmal in the ear, the Clinging (brightness) in the eye, Keeping Still in the hand, the Joyous in the mouth.

The head governs the entire body. The belly serves for storing up. The foot steps on the ground and moves; the hand holds fast. The thighs under their covering branch downward; the mouth in plain sight opens upward. The ear is hollow outside, the eye is hollow inside.

Movement and rest have their definite laws. What is easy, is easy to know; what is simple is easy to follow.

. . . the inner movement is in harmony with the environment, it can take effect undisturbed and have long duration.

It is exactly the same in the realm of action. Whatever is simple can easily be imitated. Consequently, others are ready to exert their energy in the same direction; everyone does gladly what is easy, because it is simple. The result is that energy is accumulated and the simple develops quite naturally into the manifold.

By means of the easy and the simple we grasp the laws of the whole world. When the laws of the whole world are grasped, therein lies perfection.

Looking upward, we contemplate with its help the signs in the heavens; looking down, we examine the lines of the earth. Thus we know the circumstances of the dark and the light. Going back to the beginnings of things and pursuing them to the end, we come to know the lessons of birth and of death.

The union of seed and power produces all things; the escape of the soul brings about change.

The primal powers never come to a standstill; the cycle of becoming continues uninterrruptedly.

The holy sages were able to survey all the movements under heaven. They contemplated the way in which these movements met and became interrelated, to take their course according to eternal laws.

Life leads the thoughtful person on a path of many windings. Now the course is checked, now it runs straight again.

Therefore they called the closing of the gates the Receptive, and the opening of the gate the Creative. The alternation between closing and opening they called change. The going forward and backward without ceasing they called penetration.

Therefore there is in the Changes the Great Primal Beginning. This generates the two primary forces.

Good fortune and misfortune, remorse and humiliation, come about through movement.

Good fortune and misfortune take effect through perseverance. The tao of heaven and earth becomes visible through perseverance. The tao of sun and moon becomes bright through perseverance. The movements under heaven become uniform through perseverance.

THE FORM: *List of Movements*

This numerical summary of the movements follows the paragraphs in the manual. Use it as a mnemonic while learning Tai Chi, and after it is learned as an aid for recall. Stand erect, spine straight, relax the body, and breathe deeply in and out twice—long, complete, refreshing breaths and begin.

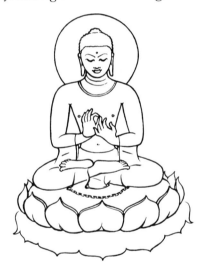

1. Homage to Buddha
2. Grasp the Swallow's Tail
3. Press Forward and Push
4. Step Up—Empty Step
5. Single Whip
6. Stork Cools Its Wings
7. Elbow Strike
8. Deflect to the Side

9. Deflect Downward
10. Parry and Punch
11. Divide Upward, Guard the Temples
12. Step Forward, Push
13. Counter-Clockwise Turn and Carry Tiger to Mountain
14. Walk Forward, Both Hands Circularly Blocking
15. Step Forward, Parry, and Punch
16. Backhand Slap
17. Repulse the Monkey, Three Retreating Steps
18. Side Pivot, Cross Wrists
19. White Crane Flying
20. Raise Left Hand, Raise Right Hand
21. Turn Directly Around and Raise the Right Hand, Then the Left
22. Grab and Pull Back
23. Step Up and Open Hand Strike
24. Draw the Bow
25. Green Dragon Step
26. Single Whip
27. Transition Step for Wave Hands Like Clouds
28. Wave Hands Like Clouds
29. Single Whip
30. Pat the Horse
31. Step Forward and Circular Block Downward
32. Side Heel Thrust Kicks, Right and Left
33. Diagonal Turn and Left Thrust Kick
34. Wind Blowing the Lotus Leaf
35. Open Palm Upward Block, with Diagonal Punch Down
36. Pivot Around, Forearm Block
37. Flying Jump Kick

38. Step In, Deflect Downward, Parry, and Punch
39. Step Back, Sweep with the Wrists
40. Circular Block and Kick with the Left Heel
41. Heel Swivel, Cross Wrists, and Pivot Around
42. Circular Block and Right Heel Kick
43. Step In, Parry, and Punch
44. Close Up, Guard the Temples
45. Press Forward and Push
46. Reverse T Step
47. Elbow Chop
48. Retreat Downward
49. Rise Up and Chop Again
50. Diagonal Single Whip
51. Wild Horse Flinging Its Mane
52. Diagonal Single Whip
53. Fair Lady Working at the Loom (Steps in Four Directions)
54. Grasp the Swallow's Tail (Variant)
55. Push Forward
56. Single Whip
57. Wave Hands Like Clouds
58. Single Whip
59. Snake Creeps Down
60. Golden Cock Stands on One Leg
61. Repulse the Monkey
62. Side Pivot, Cross Wrists
63. White Crane Flying
64. Raise Left Hand, Raise Right Hand
65. Turn Directly Around and Raise Right Hand, Then Left Hand
66. Grab and Pull Back
67. Step Up and Open Hand Strike

68. Draw the Bow
69. Deflect to the Side
70. Push and Step
71. Strike Opponent's Ears
72. Cannon Fires Through the Sky
73. Single Whip
74. Wave Hands Like Clouds
75. Single Whip
76. Water Lily Kick
77. Punch Downward
78. Step Up and Grasp the Swallow's Tail (Variant)
79. Push Forward
80. Single Whip
81. Wave Hands Like Clouds
82. Single Whip
83. Snake Creeps Down
84. Seven Star Punch
85. Retreat and Ride the Tiger
86. Slant the Body and Turn the Moon
87. Water Lily Kick
88. Shoot the Tiger
89. Grasp the Swallow's Tail
90. Push Forward
91. Step Back
92. Grasp the Swallow's Tail
93. Push Forward
94. Cross Hands and Circle Overhead

AFTERWORD

After you have been using this book to practice Kuang Ping Tai Chi, you will notice that it has taken a while to learn the Form and that there have been observable changes in your appearance and attitude. Improvement in all things, hopefully.

At this point we introduce an important variation in your practice of the Form. It would be most beneficial to relearn the entire Form in its mirror image. Although all compass points are covered by the steps, the Kuang Ping Tai Chi pattern progresses counterclockwise. We now advise you to learn the Form again, but clockwise. You would still begin facing north, but you would reverse all movements. Thus, in 1. Homage to Buddha, you would extend the right leg, having all the body's weight on the left foot, and your hand movements would reverse accordingly.

Learning the Tai Chi steps in mirror image is extremely valuable because the Form as given in this book is somewhat one-sided. Therefore, we suggest you perform the steps in reverse order to work both sides of your body equally. This reversed pattern of Tai Chi is mentally difficult—but not physically taxing. The mind rebels against it! It fights! It says: "I feel so good having learned one way, why bother working so hard to learn another way?"

This is precisely why learning the reverse pattern is challenging. It can be done quite easily—if you have the proper attitude. Practice a few movements each day. Slowly the Form develops; the resistance disappears.

Now we turn to questions from students.

Suppose my mind wanders and I can't control my thoughts during practice?

If you want to stabilize the wandering mind, try to practice Universal Post and your concentration will improve.

My movements are not flowing in a tranquil way. How can I make them smooth and flowing?

Initially, your practice will not appear relaxed, soft and quiet as you would wish, but perseverance will ultimately bring perfection and disclose the rationale of the training.

How can I use Tai Chi to defend myself?

The essential secret is never to use more than four ounces of your own strength against an opponent. As to the meanings of the techniques—how to use the movements to defend—the main ingredient is your own intuition and feeling. It is better to rely on spontaneity and not clutter the mind with endless programming, since there are so many uses for each movement. Tai Chi practice should be undertaken in the same spirit as other Buddhist/Taoist studies—that is, as an enlightenment practice to catapult you into clear, objectless awareness.

During standing practice in Universal Post, my body aches sometimes and my mind wanders. Can you recommend practices for holding the mind?

Place your tongue on the roof of your mouth—reach way back with it, toward the throat. Send mental commands throughout your body to relax, become soft. Keep your eyes half-closed and gaze out to a distance of 3 feet in front of you. Now begin to count your inhalations. Begin counting . . . one, two, three . . . to 10. Then begin again. When you can count to 10, without wandering off, your concentration will be improved and there will be quiet within your body and within your mind.

Kung Fu legends are filled with stories of male masters and feats of masculine prowess. Weren't women active?

The martial arts chroniclers and fighters have been men and therefore women's achievements and contributions have not been popularized. Chinese films often show heroines executing superb movements and quick maneuvers. They are based on old, factual stories. In China, upper-class women learned systems of self-defense. They needed them. Contemporary women are moving into Kung Fu quite easily and naturally because of their innate gracefulness. Women have always been more interested than men in the healthful aspects of life because the important function of caring for children has been mainly entrusted to them.

"Wing Chun," the system of self-defense popularized by Kung Fu's folk hero, Bruce Lee, was invented by a woman. Yim Wing Chun, whose name means "beautiful Spring," invented her set to ward off attackers without using force. She learned from a Buddhist nun, Ng Mui. This happened 400 years ago.

How much practice space do I need? I have only a small room.

When you can't go outdoors, you can practice in an area 4 feet square. That is one of the obvious things about Tai Chi as a sport. One doesn't need a special place to perform it, or special equipment or clothing. You can even perform it while traveling. It's mental Tai Chi. You can close your eyes, sit in a relaxed posture and actually see yourself performing.

How fast can I learn the Form?

People learn the Form in 10 weeks, 4 months, or longer. There is no set amount of time for learning. It's like playing a musical instrument. You play it every day.

Are there common factors to Chinese Yoga (Taoist systems) and hatha yoga (Hindu systems) ?

They are similar in that they emphasize concentration, developing mind-body controls and conscious breathing. They contain strong elements of discipline, i.e. regular practice of procedures. They all contain teachings on morality, contentment, transcendance of worldly suffering and liberation from ignorance. There are differences, too, and study reveals them.

How is Tai Chi a "spiritual" subject?

It is spiritual in the sense that by continued practice, you become acquainted with aspects of yourself that have been hidden. Your practice is devotional. By sustaining interest, by performing this personal ritual, you are performing religious acts. You are using Tai Chi as a method for integrating the material and spiritual levels of being.

How long does it take to perform the Form from beginning to end?

Performance time is variable. It can take 5 minutes to 40 minutes to do a set. The longer it takes, the better it works as exercise. By practicing slowly, you develop patience and control.

How many times should I perform the set in a day?

This is variable. No one should tell you what is the amount of food you should eat. Many people enjoy having two practice periods a day, morning and evening.

Besides the obvious physical benefits, besides the direct connection with meditation, what is the main value of Tai Chi?

This is personal and variable. Some people seek physical improvement. Of course, they may achieve this and health and longevity, too.

In the course of studying Tai Chi, it became clear that we had luckily stumbled onto a wonderful method of learning. To learn the Tai Chi method is to learn how to master structure. This is accomplished by patient, careful repetition, along with self-study. Repeat the set, and do it again and again. Soon you can see yourself moving and so you see how to proceed. Nobody has to tell you anything after a while. You have learned it.

Isn't this the way to learn everything, by careful attention?

That is the intriguing thing about Tai Chi. Once you have mastered this method for learning Tai Chi, you can apply it to anything else you wish to learn. It is infallible. It always works. Your memory improves, so all learning becomes more efficient.

Here's how it works. It uses reinforcement. With patient, daily repetition, you remember more and more and finally you see it all committed to memory. This builds inner strength. When you feel this energy, you use it for learning.

In addition to reinforcement, there is the development of steadiness. You become certain in your movements so that your attitude toward life becomes more balanced—fewer uncertainties, more confidence in decisions.

To us, the main value beyond health improvement and meditation has been psychological.

Bibliography

Arng, Lee Ying. *Chinese Leg Manoeuvres*. Honolulu: McLisa Enterprises, 1962.
———. *Lee's Modified Tai Chi for Health*. Honolulu: McLisa Enterprises, 1968.
Arng, Lee Ying, and Yen Te Hwa. *Pa Kua Chang for Self Defense*. Hong Kong: Unicorn Press, 1972.
Blofeld, John. *The Secret and Sublime, Taoist Mysteries and Magic*. New York: E. P. Dutton, 1973.
Blofeld, John. *Beyond the Gods, Buddhist and Taoist Mysticism*. New York: E. P. Dutton, 1974.
Chaudhuri, Dr. Haridas. *Philosophy of Meditation*. New York: Philosophical Library, 1965.
Chen, Y. K. *Tai Chi Chuan, Effects and Practical Applications*. Hong Kong: Unicorn Press, 1967.
Danielou, Alain. *Yoga, The Method of Re-Integration*. New York: University Books, 1955.
Gia Fu-Feng. *Tao Te Ching*. New York: Random House, 1972.
Herrigel, Eugen. *Zen and the Art of Archery*. New York: Vintage Paperback, 1971.
Huang, Al Chung-liang. *Embrace Tiger, Return to Mountain*. Moab, Utah: Real People Press, 1973.
Kuo, L. Y. *Tai Chi Chuan, Theory and Practice*. Taipeh, Taiwan. Currently in print and available from author, San Francisco.
Lu K'uan Yu. *The Secrets of Chinese Meditation*. New York: S. Weiser, 1969.
———. *Taoist Yoga, Alchemy and Immortality*. New York: S. Weiser, 1970.
———. *Ch'an & Zen Teaching* (vols. I, II, III) . New York: S. Weiser, 1962.
Minick, Michael. *The Wisdom of Kung Fu*. New York: William Morrow, 1974.
Palos, Stephan. *The Chinese Art of Healing*. New York: Bantam, 1972.
Ram Dass. *The Only Dance There Is*. Garden City, New York: Anchor Press/Doubleday, 1974.
Rawson and Legeza. *Tao, The Eastern Philosophy of Time and Change*. New York: Avon, 1973.
Smith, R. W. *Secrets of Shaolin Temple Boxing*. Rutland, Vt.: Charles E. Tuttle, 1964.
———. *Pa Kua, Chinese Boxing for Fitness and Self-Defense*. New York: Kodansha, 1967.
———. *Chinese Boxing, Methods and Masters*. Rutland, Vt.: Charles E. Tuttle, 1974.
Smith, R. W., and Cheng Man-ch'ing. *Tai Chi*. Rutland, Vt.: Charles E. Tuttle, 1967.
Tang Mong Hun. *Fundamental Exercises of Tai Chi Chuan*. Singapore: Hup Kee Press, 1966.
Wilhelm, R. *The Secret of the Golden Flower*. New York: Harcourt Brace Jovanovich, 1962.
Wilhelm, R., and Cary F. Baynes, trans. *I Ching, or Book of Changes*. Princeton: Princeton University Press, 1950.

Picture Notes

History of Kuang Ping Tai Chi

Genealogy

1. *Chen Chang Hsing—14th generation of Chen family*
2. *Yang Lu Chan*
3. *Yang Pan Hou—first son*
4. *Wong Shao Yu—lived to age 132*
5. *Kuo Lien Ying*

Master Kuo's form is patterned on the "old style" training as developed by the Chen family. Kuo's teacher, Wong Shao Yu, was the student of Yang Pan Hou. His father, Yang Lu Chan, learned under Chen Chang Hsing at a time when the training was being revised. There was the new style, or small form, and the old style, or big form. Yang Lu Chan and his first son, Pan Hou, trained according to the old style as taught by Chen Chang Hsing. Succeeding generations of Yangs trained according to the new methods. So the old style went only as far as Pan Hou. When Pan Hou was called to court to teach the Emperor and the Manchu nobles, he did not want to go, since he was loyal to the Ming Dynasty. The Manchus were not native Chinese and were considered to be foreign invaders. So Yang taught the new style, while his personal training procedures remained a closely guarded secret. He did not wish to teach his method of developing internal power to the general public, especially the Manchu nobility. Yang Lu Chan spent 18 years training under the Chens, and wanted to keep the old style training a secret. Pan Hou taught the old style set to only one person, Wong Shao Yu. Wong was put under oath not to teach as long as the Ching Dynasty lasted. He became quite a mystery figure in Peking, since it was known that he was a companion of Yang Pan Hou. When the Ching Empire fell, he was free to accept students, and selected three, out of all who applied. One of those was Kuo Lien Ying, who brought the method to San Francisco, himself becoming a living legend, until his death at age 93.

Morning Practice

Old masters recommend early morning training, before sunrise. Start the forms facing east, to take advantage of the sun's first rays. From 5-7AM the large intestine meridian is flowing. If you begin warmups, stretching, twisting and loosening up very early, you will encourage peristalsis and discharge of wastes. Start with an easy set of stretching, progressing to more advanced exercises, as shown in this book. This exercise period is most beneficial to the bones and ligaments. People are also most liable to injury at this time, so take care to perform slowly and carefully, especially if it's cold out. After 40 minutes of warming up, begin your Tai Chi forms. Try to do three or more. After Tai Chi forms, cool down with standing meditation; beginners, 10 minutes; advanced, more; but build it up gradually and slowly, to avoid straining the nervous system.

People who perform Tai Chi to strengthen their bodies and rid themselves of old injuries or diseases will feel heat and pain in the weak areas because healing energy is being transmitted. The pain and heat will eventually end, and after months of practice, the body will be strengthened and rejuvenated.

Afternoon Practice

From 11AM to 1PM, the heart meridian is flowing, so your physical level of energy, Ching, will be highest then. You won't feel stiff, aching and groggy, as in the early morning. The noon workout will strengthen and balance the mind after a morning of business or study. Start with Tai Chi warmups, slowly and carefully, as usual. Next, play Tai Chi sets. After Tai Chi sets, do Universal Post standing meditation. When you finish, you will be feeling peaceful, calm and balanced. Enjoy this state for a while, and don't rush back into mundane affairs prematurely.

114

Evening Practice

Evening practice is quite important to de-stress the mind/spirit after a busy day! As usual, do warmups first, then Tai Chi sets, then Universal Post. Don't eat for at least half an hour after practice. Never take cold drinks before or after. Please don't shock your stomach.

People with more time, interest and energy to follow the suggested training schedule will certainly derive much benefit from it. If you want to adapt it to your special needs, do so. On the other hand, you may feel it's not enough! If so, here are other special times for Taoists to pratice: full moon nights; also at midnight when the root of Yang is beginning to sprout. To strengthen your breathing, you may sit up from 3 to 5 AM and just maintain awareness of respiration. Be fully conscious of all sensations at the tip of the nose, especially the openings of the nostrils. Feel whatever sensation is presented to the awareness. Observe the changes in depth of breathing: shallow or deep. Don't try to force or change the breath in any way. When you breathe in, the air is cold. When you breathe out, it is warm. Other sensations may be itching, burning, heaviness, pain, at the nose tip. Or you may not know what you are feeling. I recommend that you focus on awareness of breathing from 3 to 5 AM, when the lung meridian is flowing. The lungs are the masters of your life force, or chi. If you can strengthen and concentrate the breathing, chi will be strengthened. If you do anything to weaken the lungs, or breathing, chi will dissipate and disperse. It's a good sign if you see a bright point of light slightly below the nostrils. That means concentration has been momentarily achieved. If you're serious about Chi Kung it will be well worth your while to cultivate at this special time. Wrap yourself up, sit cross-legged, disperse drowsiness and torpor—and consider yourself fortunate to be on the Path of the Immortals.

Advanced practitioners may wonder exactly how many Tai Chi sets to do in a day. First, you find out how many you can do comfortably, without strain, every day; then build it up a set every two months. Practice every day, with regularity. If you can do five sets a day, after two months increase to six. After two more months, add another. In this way, you keep building on plateaus. The main idea is to be sensitive to what, when, and how much you can do. It's not like loading firewood on a donkey! The training must be done joyfully, otherwise it could become a burden. It is really meditation training, so all facets must be examined meticulously. Analyze your movements minutely, so that you practice correctly.

*Let go of all negative thoughts. Anger, hatred, thoughts of violence, will keep your **Kung Fu** down, so that you can't rise to higher consciousness with it. The truth is that there aren't any opponents outside one's own laziness, ignorance, lack of discipline, and physical weakness. If you can let go of negative forces, ill will, jealousy, egotism, your **Kung Fu** will be free to rise higher and higher, without restraint. Otherwise, you hold yourself down to a lower level. Buddhists say: "Conceit is the root of all defilements." While you're training, just live in the present. Forget all worries and cares. Give yourself a mental vacation. Just breathe; no thinking. Concentrate on the movements. Be attentive to what is happening in the present. When you perform single whip, the hand goes out. Eyes and attention are on the hand all the way. Chi follows attention. Then the movements will develop real power.*

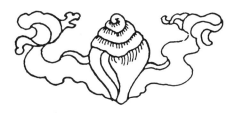

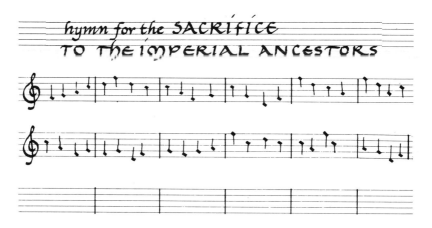

hymn for the SACRIFICE
TO THE IMPERIAL ANCESTORS

Li Po is a contemporay Taoist. Before probing the subtleties of meditation, he studied Chinese martial arts for many years. He currently resides in a remote hermitage, where he continues his study and practice of ancient ritual, amid the chirping of wild forest birds and the soundless, falling leaves.

I watch the wild, long-necked black goose
daily fly over crashing ocean
from rock to rock.

Ananda is a seeker following The Tao. Born in New York City, she now resides and works in Fort Bragg, California. She maintains private and group practice in Tai Chi, Shiatsu massage and hypnosis. She is a pioneer in integrating various disciplines for complete somatic understanding. Tai Chi Chuan conquers all enemies to peace, resulting in good will and dynamic health.

CONVENIENT ORDER FORM

WAVE HANDS LIKE CLOUDS _____ copies @ $11.95 ea. _____
For all Tai Chi lovers.

THE ESSENCE OF TAOIST MEDITATION
AND SELF MASSAGE COURSE _____ copies @ $3. ea. _____
A short instructional booklet which can improve the
present and future of your life. Clearly written and
illustrated.

THE VEGETARIAN VITALITY DIET _____ copies @ $3. ea. _____
A beautiful poster containing the most purifying raw
foods diet developed by Dr. Randolph Stone of
Polarity fame. Cures all disease.

Subtotal _____

California residents add 6% sales tax _____

Postage: add $1.50 up to $6.00
           add $2.50 over $6.00   _____

Enclosed with order, **Total** $ _____

Send Check or Money Order to:
BAMBOO PUBLISHING   P. O. Box 1037   Fort Bragg, Ca. 95437

Ship to: Name _____

           Address_____

           City _____ State _____ Zip _____

Wholesale:

Wayfarer Publications
P.O.B. 26156
Los Angeles, Ca. 90026

Bookpeople
2929 Fifth St.
Berkeley, Ca. 94710